The Complete

A TO Z

for your

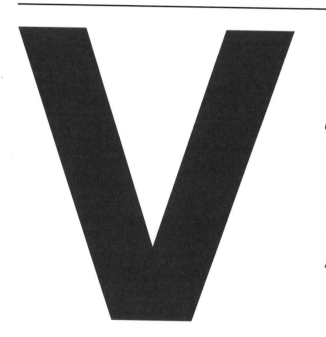

*a Women's Guide to
everything you ever
wanted to know about*
**YOUR VAGINA:
HEALTH, PLEASURE,
HORMONES,
AND MORE**

ALYSSA DWECK, M.D. *and* **ROBIN WESTEN**

FAIR WINDS

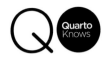

Quarto is the authority on a wide range of topics.

Quarto educates, entertains and enriches the lives of our readers—enthusiasts and lovers of hands-on living.

www.QuartoKnows.com

© 2017 Quarto Publishing Group USA Inc.
Text © 2017 Alyssa Dweck, M.D., and Robin Westen

First published in the United States of America in 2017 by
Fair Winds Press, an imprint of
Quarto Publishing Group USA Inc.
100 Cummings Center
Suite 265-D
Beverly, Massachusetts 01915-6101
Telephone: (978) 282-9590
Fax: (978) 283-2742
QuartoKnows.com
Visit our blogs at QuartoKnows.com

21 20 19 18 17   1 2 3 4 5

ISBN: 978-1-59233-767-5

Digital edition published in 2017

Library of Congress Cataloging-in-Publication Data Available

Cover Design: Burge Agency
Page Layout: Ashley Prine, Tandem Books
Illustration: Laia Albaladejo

Printed in China

This book has been written and published strictly for informational purposes, and in no way should it be used as a substitute for consultation with professional therapists or physicians. All facts in this book came from scientific publications, personal interview, published trade books, self-published materials by experts, magazine articles, and the personal practice experiences of the authorities quoted or sources cited. This book does not create a doctor patient relationship. The author and publisher are providing you with information in this work so that you can have the knowledge and can choose, at your own risk, to act on that knowledge.

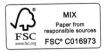

To Evan, the brains behind the operation

—Alyssa Dweck, M.D.

To Howie—always

—Robin Westen

Contents

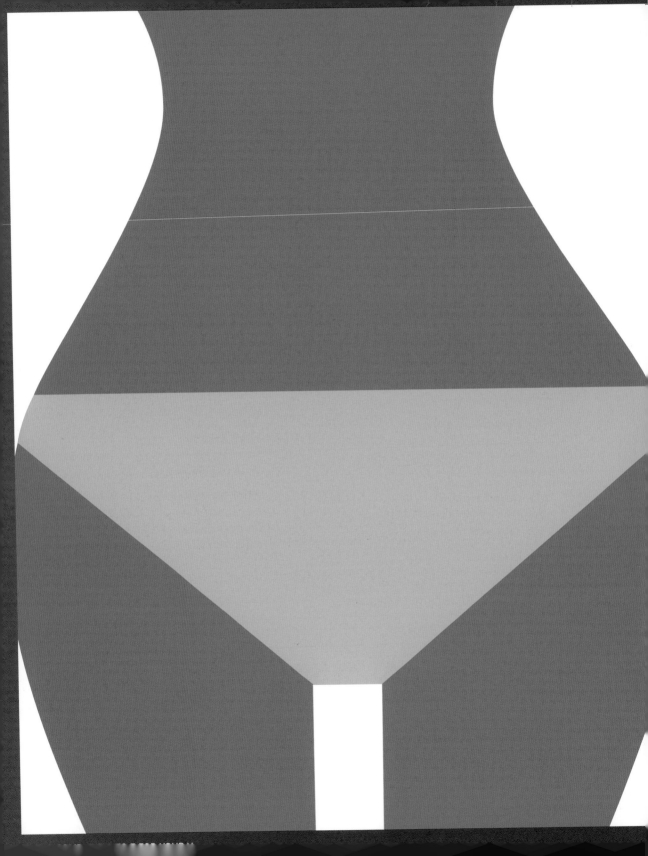

FOREWORD

What is it about the word *VAGINA*? In some circles, specifically prime time TV and news outlets, the word *vagina* is either banned completely or its use is significantly limited. For reasons unbeknown to me, saying *vagina* is at times considered offensive, inappropriate, vulgar, dirty, or profane. I am a gynecologist. I "speak vagina" all day every day. I speak vagina at work, in public, and even at the dinner table. To me, a vagina is just a body part similar to an arm, leg, mouth, or nose.

I have seen thousands of vaginas, and what I have come to realize over the years is this: Women really want to know, am I normal down there? They are curious, interested, excited, elated, petrified, mortified, tearful, or panic-stricken in their need to know what's normal and what's not. Women seek reassurance, guidance, and comraderie when it comes to the vagina. Chances are, that's why you're reading this right now.

Truth be told, I get Facebooked regularly, stopped in the grocery store weekly, and sidelined in the gym daily by friends, acquaintances, and even strangers who know my profession; they all have questions and concerns about their vaginas. Some issues are straightforward. Others? Not so much. But one thing is certain. When I speak vagina, women listen attentively. They eavesdrop or gather around to hear the latest vag news. That is why I *had* to write this book. I want to speak vagina to the masses, demystify it, and remove the taboo surrounding the subject.

Rather than talking yeast infections in the produce aisle or labiaplasty on the treadmill, I want to get the word out far and wide, to educate women in an easy-to-read, nonthreatening, and direct way. I want to share medically sound and up-to-date information, and I want to have a little fun while I do it.

So, here it is: a humorous but informative guide to the sometimes mysterious and always amazing VAGINA! Some of the chapters ahead are more "medical" than others, but they all involve the V. There are chapters that may embarrass some and might even offend others, but rest assured, all information stems from the experiences I have been fortunate enough to share with my patients over the years—experiences I think most women can benefit from.

Please read, laugh, and learn. Let's speak vagina!

—Alyssa Dweck, MS, MD, FACOG

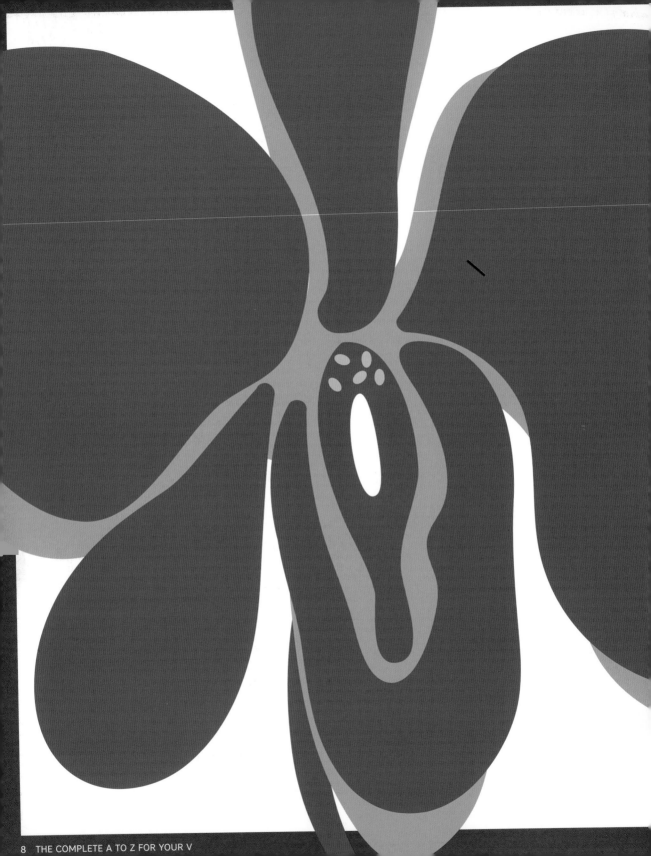

Let's have a party— the vajayjay's coming out!

INTRODUCTION

Our Vs: They're the subject of girl talk over coffee, blabbed about on *Veep*, discussed by Chelsea Handler, described on *Broad City*, joked over on *Real Time with Bill Maher*, rapped on by Lil Wayne, mocked in *Date Night*, enjoyed on *Girls*, painted on canvases, represented in caves, sculpted into walls, monologued on Broadway, banned, beautified, deified, pierced, waxed, creamed, oiled, stretched, tightened, tattooed, glorified, despised, and mythologized. There are over a thousand slang words for them: who-ha, vajayjay, cha cha, lady flower, foo foo, cooch, noonie, love clam, twinkle, love canal, the great gorge, pink, pussy, salmon canyon, and oasis, to name just a few. You can order mugs, t-shirts, songs, poems, pens, pencils, posters, and magnets with the word *vagina* in, over, or on them. After generations of the whole subject being taboo, lady parts are experiencing a fabulous renaissance in which people are beginning to talk openly and freely about their bits, their experiences, their health, and their rights.

Culture isn't the only thing that's changing in the world of vaginas. Suddenly there seems to be a market for putting the va-va-voom back in the vajayjay. Procedures that tighten the V, sculpt the labia, or restore the hymen comprise the fastest-growing area of cosmetic surgery in the United States, up by 70 percent from 2015 to 2016. Spas in New York, LA, DC, and elsewhere offer "vagina rejuvenation," which can mean irrigating the vaginal passage, slipping in a "breath" mint, massaging the clit in order to boost its sensitivity, or applying a tightening cream promising to reduce the vagina's appearance to a "youthful" state for a full 24 hours. (Think: Cinderella having a ball!) There's also Gwyneth Paltrow's suggestion to steam-clean your vagina, and then there are lasers and radiofrequency devices promising cures for loose vaginas, discoloration, and more. We could go on . . . and on . . .

Yet, despite all the attention, most of us know squat about our salmon canyon. For example, Summer's Eve, a women's hygiene company, surveyed women from all backgrounds across America and found that nearly 70 percent of respondents could not identify five major parts of their female genitalia, and nearly 60 percent struggled with unresolved feelings just about the word *vagina*.

Need more evidence that when it comes to our lovely V's we're in the dark but want and need to be brought to light? Consider these stats from the Association of Reproductive Health Professionals:

- While women perform breast self-exams regularly, only half (49 percent) of the survey respondents have ever performed a self-exam of their vagina. Twenty-four percent have not looked at their vagina in a year or longer. How sad.

- Two-thirds of the women (65 percent) surveyed agree that vaginal health and research have not received the proper attention they deserve. Agreed.

- More than half of the women surveyed (59 percent) concur that society has too many misconceptions about vaginas. Totally.

- Ninety percent of the survey respondents agree that it's important for women to be sufficiently educated about the vagina. Hello . . . That's why I'm here.

- Nearly three in four women surveyed (73 percent) believe that the vagina is still a shocking topic. Gulp.

- Some women consider their vaginas as "ugly," "gross," "dirty," and "embarrassing." Let me say this right now—this has got to stop!

- Only half of the women surveyed (51 percent) consider themselves to be extremely/very knowledgeable about their vaginas. Let's change that!

> *Just as women's bodies are softer than men's, so their understanding is sharper.*
>
> —Christine de Pisan

The good news is this: Times are changing fast and furiously. First, I've found in my practice that more women are willing to talk to me about issues that are affecting them during and after menopause. And that's a plus. Also, in the past few years, women have had to deal with plenty of new and different issues, including infections from the oh-so-popular, bare-it-all Brazilian wax, piercings gone awry, tattoos run amok, and irritation from speed-breaking spinning classes. There's been new thinking on estrogen replacement, and a controversial vaccine (though less so these days as studies show it doesn't promote "promiscuity"—ugh, that word!) to protect young girls from HPV (human papillomavirus, or cervical warts). In fact, the newest version, Gardasil 9, covers the most common strains of HPV, and it's even been mandated for all middle school–aged girls in Virginia. Plus, there's the redesign of tampons (some infused with herbs) and pads, the new and rage-worthy DivaCup, a host of new and ultra-titillating sex toys, "go-commando" panty liners, the vajazzling craze, reconsideration on vitamins and soy, new treatments for vulvodynia (the vaginal pain syndrome thousands of women suffer from), and so much more. There's even a rumor that sex researchers have discovered the A-spot, which some claim one-ups the G-spot for guaranteeing over-the-top O pleasure. This may be more myth than fact, as research on it is as scanty as a thong. Moving higher up on our pleasure radar is the latest fascination with "squirting," (aka female ejaculation) even though a recent study in the *Journal of Sexual Medicine* says the little burst of liquid is probably nothing more than pee.

If some of these things sound utterly unfamiliar, worry not! This book is going to tell absolutely all. Women crave the inside scoop on their quims—rightfully so. Maybe that's why Google has over 21 million entries for *vagina*. We want to be in on the latest everything about everything, from self-exams, tampons, Pap tests, cunnilingus, allergies, birth, yeast infections, and semen allergies, to ingrown pubic hairs, Kegels, lubricants, and more . . . much more. The Internet, unfortunately, often leads you to scary places filled with misinformation written by people who have pretty much zero clue what they're talking about. My aim is to give you the facts—up-to-date and judgment free.

Dear Kitty:

I'd like to ask Peter whether he knows what girls look like down there. I don't think boys are as complicated as girls. You can easily see what boys look like in photographs or pictures of male nudes, but with women, it's different. In women, the genitalia, or whatever they're called, are hidden between their legs. . . .

—Anne Frank's Diary

THE V THROUGHOUT HISTORY

But first things first. Let's take a look through the cultural kaleidoscope, from today's fad of focusing on smaller labias and almost infantile vulvas to the big bush being the in hairdo to the big bush being so far out, from neo vaginas for those born without one to the trans population. There are so many different kinds of vaginas in the world, and the way the V is portrayed in society, art, literature, pornography, and elsewhere reflects those variations—though you might not be able to tell that from some of the more pervasive porn out there today. That said, everybody begins with the vagina in some way: You were conceived and born, right? Or, as Catherine Blackledge, author of the comprehensive *The Story of V*, writes, "The vagina is the seat of female sexual pleasure, the site of the creation of humankind and the channel for its birth."

Self-proclaimed feminist author Naomi Wolf sees our cha cha from a historical perspective: "The way we understand and envision the vagina at certain moments in history is a metaphor for how we are willing to see women in general and how women are encouraged to see themselves. From the Greeks and the Romans to Freud, from pornography and health to goddesses, from worship to denigration and even mutilation, there is a history of this wonderful organ, the 'dark continent' of female sexuality, well deserving of its own story."

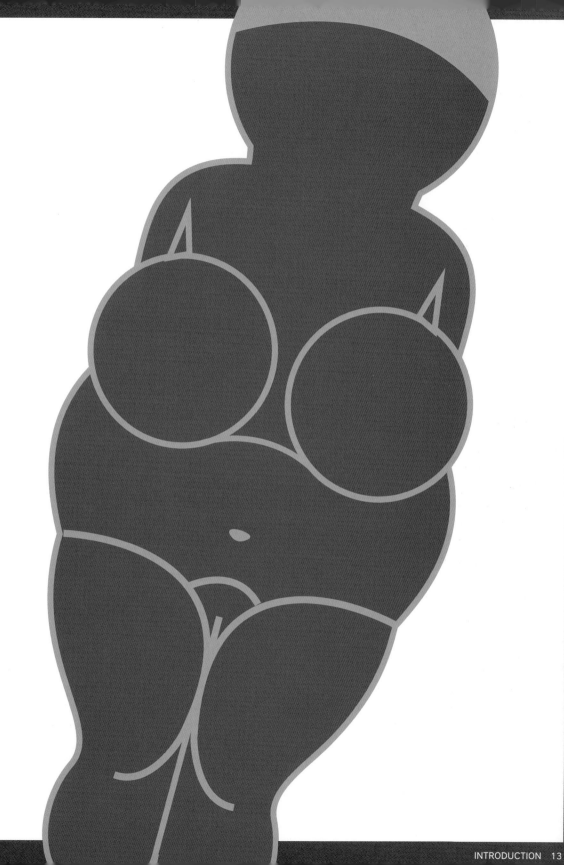

> *This to my mind is the vagina as icon, sacred, inviolable, worshipped. The sister and source from which all human life springs.*
>
> —Catherine Blackledge

True, the historical, artistic, and literary record of our who-ha ranges from awesome to alarming, mirroring our culture's view of sexuality. Before the nineteenth century, terms for the V were affectionate and kind. Even the word *cunt*, one of the oldest words for female genitalia, was meant to mean something warm and cuddly. In fact, before the fifteenth century, cunt was just another word, so much a part of everyday vocabulary that it was used in naming public streets. Around 1230, for example, there was a London street called Gropecunt Lane, and in Paris there was a rue Grattecon, which translates as Scratchcunt Street. But after the fifteenth century, cunt was totally taboo. In England it was forbidden in speech and print and a legal offense to publish the word.

Vagina (what!) . . . vagina (what!) . . . I want to have sex with your vagina (uhh) Vagina (what!) . . . vagina (what!) . . . What time is it? It's vagina.

—Jon Lajoie, "E=MC Vagina"

But get this: The much tamer word *vagina* (although recently seen and heard in ads for issues such as vaginal dryness and painful sex) is rarely used in the United States in commercials, even when the product being hawked is a tampon! Thank goodness this uptight, V-dissing perspective isn't the whole story. In fact, throughout history, cultures all over the world have at times celebrated the gorgeous, glorious lady flower. Vagina art can be found in archaic statuettes, amulets, and figurines as well as carved on seals and jewelry and in sculptures, installations, and paintings in our modern museums.

During the Paleolithic period, images of vulvas were emblazoned on various Stone Age sites in France, Spain, and Russia, as well as other locations. Perhaps one of the most striking representations of the V can be seen on the walls of a cave in Vienne, France. Here, a remarkable trinity of vulvas was carved on the rock surface as far back as 17,000 years ago.

Moving along, in 1896 German archeologists discovered a temple site in Turkey dating back to the fifth century BCE. Within it were seven petite terra-cotta females. What makes them so fantabulous is the artist created these little sculptures so that the face, stomach, and genitals merge into one image. Indeed they are, without dispute, total vulva women.

But these little gals don't take the proverbial Honey Pot Award for most outstanding vulva. That goes to a figurine dating from between 23,000 and 21,000 BCE, carved out of limonite and found in southern France. This Venus figurine displays a huge curved oval vulva that is slit right down the center.

Some of the oldest examples of skirt-lifting and vulva-revealing images date from 1400 BCE and are found on a Syrian cylinder seal. On it, viewers can easily see three women either spreading their legs wide or lifting their clothes to reveal, with pride and without prejudice, their impressive V's.

Historians say it's amazing that these kinds of "vaginic" works of art survived considering by the seventeenth century so many were ordered to be destroyed, buried, or burned. Thank you very much, England.

African culture was slow to condemn V exposure. As recently as the twentieth century, a common gesture in some African societies was to expose the vulva as if to shame someone, saying, "Hey, don't forget where you came from, buddy."

In other parts of the world, vulvas created by natural rock formations are still venerated. For instance, in Japan, parents encourage their children to play near rocks that resemble genitals. Especially renowned is a group of formations in Kyushu. It's believed these shapes offer good luck and health to anyone who is within their vicinity. The same goes in Thailand on the island of Koh Samui. There, two natural vulva rock formations in the cliffs overlooking the sea are used as a place not only of prayer, but of pilgrimage as well. Tourists who visit the sexy formations in the morning hours will see native Thais leaving flower offerings on the sacred spot.

The Sanskrit word for vagina is *yoni*, meaning womb, origin, source, and universe. And let's not forget the V-loving ancient Egyptians. They focused on the downward-pointing triangle shape and made it the symbol of sacred creativity. Perhaps that's why the entrance to the queen's chamber in the pyramid of Cheops is indicated by a downward-pointing triangle. BTW: If you could exam it, the same triangle is seen in the interior structure of the uterus. And, not to be left out, Tantric lore also expresses the vagina as the entrance to the past as well as the future.

Speaking of interior views, the famous Taoist text "The Wondrous Discourse of Su Nü" explains how vaginas come in eight varieties and sizes. From smallest to largest, the eight are known as:

- The Zither, or Lute String

- The Water-caltrop Teeth, or Water-chestnut Teeth

- The Peaceful Valley, or Little Stream

- The Dark, or Mysterious Pearl

- The Valley Seed, or Valley Proper

- The Palace of Delight, or Deep Chamber

- The Inner Door, or Gate of Prosperity

- The North Pole

Reinier de Graaf, who was a brilliant seventeenth-century Dutch physician, anatomist, and admirer of the V, made major discoveries in reproductive biology. He was effusive and poetic about the vagina's ability to be the perfect hostess. Get this:

> The woman's vagina is so cleverly constructed that it will accommodate itself to each and every penis; it will go out to meet a short one, retire before a long one, dilate for a fat one, and constrict for a thin one. Nature has taken account of every variety of penis. There's no need to solicitously seek a scabbard the same size as your knife. . . . Every man can thus come together with every woman and every woman with every man.

With this understanding in mind, that vaginas can accommodate so many penis sizes, is it surprising vibrators took off at home as well as in the doc's office? While this easy matching of anatomy sizes might lead one to think that there is plenty of penis-provided satisfaction going around, let's face it, the big O isn't always (or even usually) about the penis. Even in the uptight United States, as early as the 1890s, women could purchase a $5 portable vibrator advertised as "perfect for weekend trips." This soon supplanted paying a doctor $2 a visit for

him to stimulate the clitoris until an orgasm was reached. Yeah, it was really done to "cure hysteria" (what was once thought to be a nervous disease in women, stemming from their baby makers, with the root word, *hystera*, being Greek for "womb"). Hmmm . . . not sure if that would be covered under health insurance today.

Sadly though, in some cultures, there's no celebration of the V's versatility and ability to feel pleasure. Whether it's called female genital cutting, female circumcision, female genital mutilation, or clitorectomy, it's a surgical procedure ranging from drawing blood to removing the clitoris by itself to removing the external genitals and joining the sides to leave only a small opening. This horrendous practice dates to ancient times; usually performed on young girls and in a ritual context, it is purported by its practitioners to guard a girl's virginity and reduce her sexual desires. Because it is usually undertaken in unhygienic conditions, even today, cutting may lead to severe bleeding, infection, debilitating pain, and death. The long-term consequences of this barbaric practice can include an inability to urinate or expel menstrual blood, pain during sexual intercourse, and prolonged childbirth—not to mention the psychological and social trauma that may linger.

CELEBRATING THE V

Rather than ending this section on a sad note, let's celebrate our amazing cha cha by exploring modern literary and art works. This book would not be complete without giving kudos to Eve Ensler, author of the iconic work *The Vagina Monologues*. Ensler brought the vagina out of the genital closet by interviewing a diverse group of more than 200 women about their vaginas: young and old, married and single; heterosexual, bisexual, and lesbian; working-class women, professional women, and sex workers; women of various races. When Ensler performs the monologues, she does some of them verbatim, some as composites, and some are her invented impressions. The subjects, which all have to do with vaginas, include such topics as what a vagina looks like, what goes in and comes out of vaginas, menstruation and birth, and more playfully, "If your vagina got dressed, what would it wear?" or "If your vagina could talk, what would it say, in two words?"

Feminist artist Judy Chicago did fabulous work breaking the vagina visual art barrier in her piece *The Dinner Party*, an installation of ceramic vagina place settings representing 39 mythical and historical famous women, which she produced from 1974 to 1979. Despite art world resistance to her vagina theme, it toured sixteen venues in six countries on three continents to a viewing audience of one million. Since 2007 it has been on permanent exhibition at the Brooklyn Museum in New York City.

More recently, there's the quim work by Brighton, UK, artist Jamie McCartney. McCartney convinced more than 400 women, aged 18 to 76, to spread their legs so that he could make a plaster cast of their vaginas and vulvas and display them en masse. McCartney's socially conscious installation was five years in the making. Included in his piece are mothers and daughters, identical twins, trans men and women, as well as a woman pre- and postnatal, and another one pre- and post-labioplasty. McCartney's work uses shock, humor, and spectacle ultimately educating people about what normal women really look like.

HALLELUJAH!

HOW MUCH DO YOU KNOW ABOUT YOUR V?

TEST YOUR V KNOWLEDGE

1. How many ladies don't have an orgasm with intercourse alone?
   a. 10 percent
   b. 50 percent
   c. 75 percent

2. Who discovered the G-spot?
   a. Walt Disney. Ha-ha. It's make-believe.
   b. Helen Gurley Brown
   c. Ernst Grafenberg, a German gynecologist

3. Why is it okay to have sex during pregnancy?
   a. You wouldn't be horny if it wasn't.
   b. The baby is protected within the uterus, cushioned by fluid.
   c. It's not okay! Abstain!

4. The morning-after pill is
   a. a great contraceptive.
   b. a treatment to prevent pregnancy after unprotected sex.
   c. only a dream.

5. Yeast infections can be caused by
   a. wearing panty liners.
   b. taking antibiotics.
   c. both of the above.

6. What can you do if you think your labia is too "fat"?
   a. Consider (carefully) labioplasty.
   b. Do special labia exercises and/or go on a diet and you'll lose weight down there, too.
   c. Love it and leave it alone, because labias come in many shapes and sizes.

7. What is the "transition zone"?
   a. The end of fertility and the start of menopause
   b. An area of the cervix where squamous and glandular cells meet
   c. A one-way ticket to incredible orgasms

8. Who doesn't need a Pap smear (aka Pap test)?
   a. Women who are younger than 16 and have not had sexual intercourse
   b. Most women between the ages of 30 and 40
   c. Women who have had a hysterectomy and kept their cervix

9. What are vulvar skin tags?
   a. A potential sign of cancer. See your doctor immediately.
   b. Outgrowths of normal skin. No worries.
   c. Smooth white bumps under the surface of your vulva's skin.

10. What's a common cause of low sex drive?
   a. Sugar
   b. Exercise
   c. Poor body image

11. What helps reduce the pain after a bikini wax?
   a. Staying pale down there for 24 hours before and after the procedure (meaning no tanning booths or sun exposure)
   b. Wearing Spanx
   c. Getting weekly waxes

12. What's the most popular place to pierce the vagina?
   a. Inner labia
   b. Clitoral hood
   c. Outer labia

13. Who put vaginal steaming on the radar?
   a. Carrie Bradshaw
   b. Gwyneth Paltrow
   c. Lady Gaga

14. To keep your lady flower lovely, you should
   a. douche frequently.
   b. take bubble baths.
   c. wear cotton underwear (or "go commando").

15. Can women get addicted to porn?
   a. No way!
   b. Yes! Duh.
   c. Porn addiction in women is rare.

16. Both gonorrhea and chlamydia are treated with
   a. antibiotics.
   b. douching.
   c. abstinence.

17. What can relieve menstrual cramps?
   a. Chocolate
   b. Sex
   c. Aerobics

18. Many women going through menopause experience
   a. hot flashes.
   b. cramps.
   c. weight loss.

19. A woman trying to get pregnant should have intercourse
   a. on days 1 to 4 of a 28-day cycle.
   b. on day 14 only of a 28-day cycle.
   c. depending on the woman's cycle length, every other day on and around ovulation, approximately days 10 to 19.

20. Tampons have been linked to which of the following diseases?
   a. HIV
   b. Toxic shock syndrome
   c. Cervical cancer

21. Which is a leading cause of infertility?
    a. Sexually transmitted diseases
    b. Psychological problems
    c. Lack of physical activity

22. If you notice a pinpoint hole in your diaphragm, you should
    a. plug it up with contraceptive gel.
    b. get a new diaphragm.
    c. do nothing—it's unlikely that sperm will get through.

23. During perimenopause, you should continue using some sort of contraception
    a. until you skip a period.
    b. until it's been a full year without your period.
    c. You don't need birth control during perimenopause.

24. The following is true about HPV:
    a. You are fully protected from transmission by using a condom.
    b. It is an uncommon virus, and you're unlikely to get it.
    c. In most instances, HPV will not lead to cervical cancer.

25. A colposcopy is
    a. a form of birth control.
    b. a microscopic exam of the cervix to check for abnormal cells.
    c. a new gynecological app for your iPhone.

26. A Bartholin's cyst can be treated in all of the following ways except
    a. warm soaks, pain medication, and drainage.
    b. leaving it alone; it may go away by itself.
    c. having a lot of sex so that it will pop.

27. You can prevent a urinary tract infection by all of the following ways except
    a. wiping from front to back after going to the bathroom.
    b. holding in your urine all day.
    c. urinating before and after sex.

True or False

28. Vaginal discharge is always a yeast infection.
    (T) (F)

29. Low libido has only one cause, low hormone levels, and a simple hormone pill will cure it.
    (T) (F)

30. Bleeding from the rectum is always due to hemorrhoids; evaluation is not needed.
    (T) (F)

31. You can get genital herpes from having oral sex.
    (T) (F)

32. The birth control pill offers protection against ovarian and uterine cancers.
    (T) (F)

YOUR V SCORE

Give yourself five points for each correct answer. Then total the score and read your analysis below to find out how much you really know about all things V!

ANSWERS

1. C	14. C	27. B
2. C	15. B	28. F
3. B	16. A	29. F
4. B	17. B	30. F
5. C	18. A	31. T
6. A/C	19. C	32. T
7. B	20. B	
8. A	21. A	
9. B	22. B	
10. C	23. B	
11. A	24. C	
12. B	25. B	
13. B	26. A	

IF YOU SCORED BETWEEN 140 AND 160 POINTS:

Congratulations, Sister! You have above-average knowledge about your V as well as other areas of your femme health. This will not only serve your physical, emotional, and sexual needs, but will probably make you the go-to confidante to all your girlfriends who are feeling a little unsure about their lady flower. But hold that bouquet! Sometimes being a know-it-all keeps women away from appointments they should make, especially an annual examination with their gynecologist. A smart, well-read, and savvy woman like you should remember to seek help when a problem arises. It's the perfect way to put your V-knowledge to good use.

IF YOU SCORED BETWEEN 90 AND 135 POINTS:

You have basic V-knowledge, and that's one of the reasons why you take such good care of your cha cha and your other feminine health needs. But there are certain areas that can use a little more know-how. Go over your answers and find out where your smarts are shortchanged. Then look through the book to fill in the blanks and to get a better picture of what's going on down there. You've got potential to really grasp not only the fundamentals but also the finer points of female health. If you still have questions, don't be shy. Talk them over with your gynecologist until you get a deeper understanding. It's your body, after all.

IF YOU SCORED UNDER 85 POINTS:

For you, it's pretty much a mystery down there. But if it helps you feel better about your low score, realize you're not alone. Lots of women are in the dark when it comes to their vagina, and that's really a pity because it's such a fantastic part of you. You might have been brought up to feel shy or ashamed about your cha cha; it was not something discussed in your home or among your girlfriends. Even when you go to the doctor, you remain in the dark and never ask questions. Well, it's time to change all that! Open these pages and read on. You'll not only learn what's going on in the land of your V, but you also might be able to leave self-consciousness behind . . . or at least take a few steps in that direction.

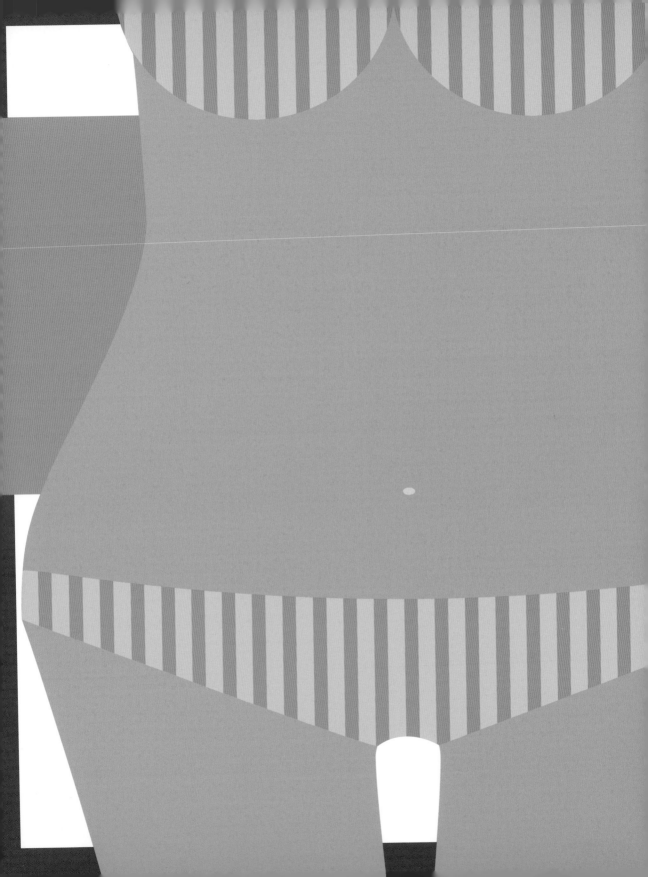

Your

V

from

A to Z

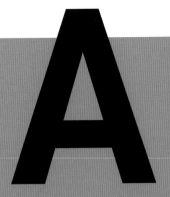

A

IS FOR THE A-SPOT

A- and G-Spots and Every
Erogenous Zone You've Ever Imagined!
Plus O's, O's, and More O's!

Isn't it enough we're supposed to be the most awesome girlfriends, amazing moms, devoted wives, fantastic friends, career-climbing professionals, and creative house organizers—now we're supposed to be XXX porn stars? At least that's how it can feel in our culture because of how women are often portrayed in the media. Hey, if you want to be a porn star, do it. No judgments! But whether you do or not, here's the thing, girlfriend, you want to have a good (hey, make that hot, sexy, transcendental) time in bed. Otherwise, well, you might not only get bored right out of the bedroom, you could end up resenting your partner as well. And no one wants that. So, let's get down and dirty, cover the basics, and then rev up your erogenous zones.

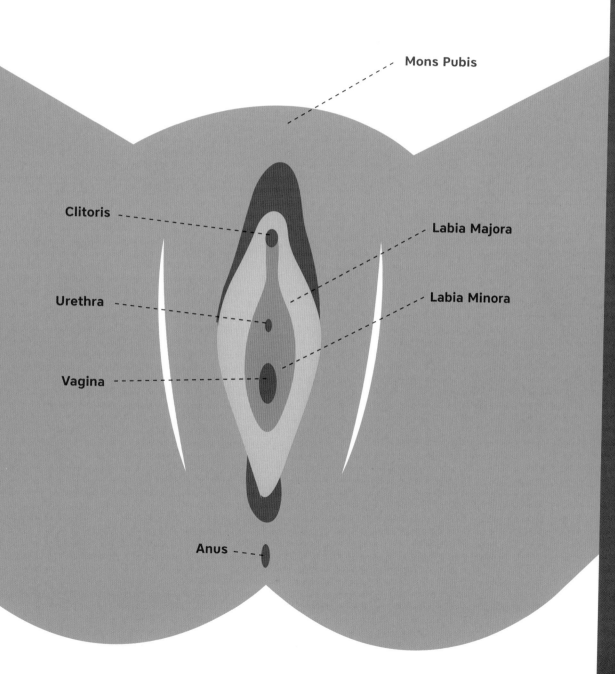

Mons Pubis

Clitoris

Labia Majora

Urethra

Labia Minora

Vagina

Anus

> *A woman's orgasm is such a fragile thing, dependant as much upon her mind as on her clitoris.*
>
> —Megan Hart, Author

WHAT EXACTLY IS AN ORGASM?

Let's put it this way: When you're having one, you probably won't hear the dryer ringing, traffic in the background, the dog whimpering to go out, or your neighbors arguing. But let's start with foreplay, where the most satisfying lovemaking sessions begin. That warm, all is well with the world feeling you're hopefully experiencing during foreplay is the rush of blood moving straight to your vajayjay and clit. Without getting too techie—and ruining the mood—it's around this time the walls of your vagina start to secrete beads of lubrication that eventually get bigger and bigger and flow together. If that doesn't happen easily, no problemo—hello, helpful LUBE.

Onward: As you get hotter, blood continues to flood your pelvic area; your breathing speeds up, heart rate increases, nipples get erect, and the lower part of your V narrows so that it can grip the penis (if that's what's in there—it could be a finger, dildo, or vibrator; tongue, anyone?). If all goes swimmingly, a lovely amount of nerve and muscle tension builds in your genitals, pelvis, buttocks, and thighs—until yippee! your body involuntarily releases all at once in a series of intensely pleasurable waves. Voilà! Your orgasm!

Oh, girlfriend, if only life were always so easy breezy.

I'M ALMOST THERE . . . ABOUT TO PEAK . . . AND THEN I LOSE MOMENTUM. WHAT'S GOING ON?

Nine times out of ten it's because you're probably not getting enough clitoral stimulation. You'll get close to orgasm, and your partner (or it could be you if you're masturbating) changes what he or she is doing. Or it could all be in your head. The fact is, for a woman, the largest erogenous zone is her brain. I mean, if you're thinking it's not going to happen, or you're wondering whether you got that email you've been waiting for, you might as well kiss an orgasm good-bye.

FROM THE AS-IF-YOU-NEED-ANOTHER-REASON FILES Sex is a beauty treatment! Scientific tests find that when women make love, they produce the hormone estrogen, which makes hair shine and skin smooth.

THE LOWDOWN ON LUBRICANTS

Not all lubes are the same. Like most things in life, each has its plusses and minuses. Try them out, talk to friends, or speak with your health care pro for a recommendation.

Water-Based	Silicone	Oil-Based	Hybrid
• Thick	• Slippery	• Thick	• Mostly water /some silicone
• Easy to wash off	• Long lasting	• Avoid petroleum	• Slick
• Short-lasting, needs reapplications	• Water insoluble	• Incompatible with latex condoms	• Thick
• Sticky	• Might stain sheets	Popular Choice: Coconut Oil	• Compatible with latex condoms
• Compatible with latex condoms	• Incompatible with silicone toys		• Generally compatible with silicone toys
Popular brands: Astroglide, KY Jelly	• Compatible with latex condoms		Popular Brand: SLIQUID™
	Popular brand: Überlube Wet Platinum		

WHY YOU MAY NOT BE HAVING AN ORGASM—FOR REAL

There may be medically oriented reasons why your O is so ellusive:

- As mentioned before, not enough (or any) clitoral stimulation. What to do? Change position, try a vibrator, or educate your partner on where to touch you.

- Menopause = less: less estrogen, less vaginal/vulvar blood supply, less natural lubrication, and (as if that's not enough, or less than enough) it takes longer to orgasm and there may be pain. See page 73 for solutions.

- Neurological probs such as herniated disc in the lumbosacral (lower back) area, diabetes, or multiple sclerosis.

- Diminished blood supply because of chronic diseases like hypertension, heart disease, and diabetes.

- Meds—specifically but not limited to SSRI antidepressants.

TRUE OR FALSE? THERE IS JUST ONE EROGENOUS ZONE.

Oh, so very false! An erogenous zone is any area of your body that has heightened sensitivity, and the stimulation of it results in the production of sexual thrills! Women (and guys, too) have erogenous zones all over their bodies. But what turns one gal on may be a total turn-off to someone else—sort of like ice cream flavors. Clit, eyelids, eyebrows, temples, shoulders, hands, arms, feet, hair, lips, neck, nipples, breasts, navel, thighs, wrists, behind the knees, hands . . . shall we go on? No, let your partner go on.

FACTOID If you're not reaching the big O while having intercourse, you're not alone. About 75 percent of girlfriends never have a climax that way. We need a little help from our friend. Who's that friend? It could be a toy, hands, a tongue, or something even more creative. O no: Around 10 to 15 percent of women have never experienced a climax.

ABOUT 1 PERCENT OF WOMEN can orgasm solely through breast stimulation. If you're one of them, you're a lucky lady! Other women who hit the sexual jackpot? Those who report over-the-moon-and-stars nocturnal orgasms (O'ing while sleeping) without any obvious tactile or manual stimulation.

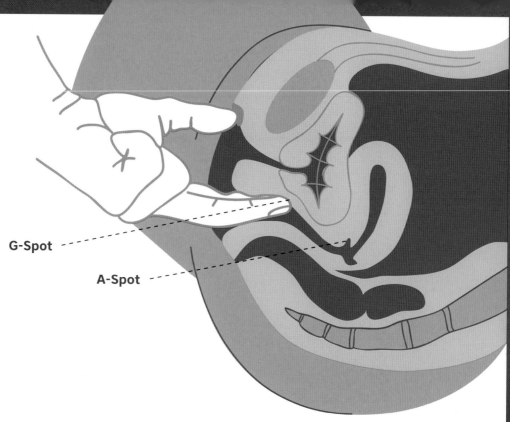

G-Spot

A-Spot

WHAT'S THIS ABOUT THE G-SPOT?

If you're asking, it probably means you haven't found yours—yet! So let me get down to a little background and then the instructions. The G-spot is not an agreed upon actual anatomic structure in traditional medical literature. However, for those who believe, the G-spot (some folks call it the urethral sponge) is wrapped around your urethra. When you're getting hot and bothered, the G-spot swells with fluid and the juices push into your vagina where they're felt on the V wall. And, honey, it feels great! The best way to stimulate the G-spot is through rhythmic massage with fingers, a penis, or dildo. It may take your partner some practice to locate it. Plus, it might take some practice for you to connect with your G-spot and learn how to experience the vaginal orgasms (which aren't nearly as common as clitoral orgasms) that are accompanied by its stimulation. But oh baby baby—it's so worth it.

Q. What's the difference between a golf ball and a G-spot?
A. A man will spend two hours searching for a golf ball.

SO, CAN I FIND THE G-SPOT MYSELF?

Sure, it's not hard to find. Just insert your index or middle finger into your vagina with your palm facing upward. You might have to use your middle finger if your G-spot is located farther up the front wall. Once your finger is inside, make a "come here" motion with it—and that should pretty much do it.

THE A-SPOT

The existence of the "A-spot" is even more questionable when you look in traditional medical literature, however, many women believe in the anterior fornix, a spot on the front wall of the vagina a few inches past the G-spot, and it's rumored to induce orgasm. For your partner to reach it, you'll need to have your hips propped up on a pillow, move into missionary position, and thrust high during intercourse. Credibility alert: Some folks say the A-spot is a whole lot a hooey.

WHENEVER I HAVE A G-SPOT ORGASM, IT FEELS LIKE I'M PEEING.

My dear sister, you may have ejaculated, or yes indeed, you may have "peed." Beverly Whipple, who is an American sex guru and co-author of the original G-spot book, says that a vaginal orgasm may produce ejaculate—as much as about half a coffee cupful. A recent study in the *Journal of Sexual Medicine* suggests that female ejaculate has the same chemical makeup as urine, and thus perhaps it is just that. The jury is still out on this, but an intense fascination with the issue exists nonetheless. What is certainly true is that some women leak a little urine during sex. However, when urine leaks during sex, it's often during foreplay or vigorous intercourse, rather than during orgasm.

FROM THE EVERYONE-HAS-AN-OPINION FILES

For women the best aphrodisiacs are words. The G-spot is in the ears. He who looks for it below there is wasting his time.

—Isabel Allende

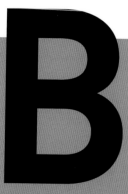

B

IS FOR BABY, OOOH BABY, BABY

Your Body (and Your Sex Life!)
During Pregnancy and Postpartum

If you've ever doubted for one itsy-bitsy second whether your vajayjay was truly wondrous, just think about the truly astounding feat of giving birth. If you've ever given birth, you really know what I'm talking about. Amazing, right? Yes, but also complicated. So let's get a good look at what happens to your lovely hothouse flower when you have a baby. And while we're at it, we'll also see why it can cause your sex drive to go on a chilly hiatus.

Giving birth is like taking your lower lip and forcing it over your head.

—Carol Burnett

CAN I HAVE SEX WHILE I'M PREGNANT?

You're not alone if you're worrying about whether it's safe to have sexual intercourse during pregnancy. Just know this: Sex is not harmful. Unless your doctor has nixed the idea, you can have sex throughout the entire nine months. Whether or not you actually want to have intercourse at any point during a pregnancy is the real story. And if you don't feel like it, sweetie, then don't. There may be times when having sex is physically uncomfortable because of your changing shape. If you're motivated (read: horny!), you can experiment to find which positions are easiest and feel the best for whatever stage you're in. Commonly recommended positions, especially for the later term, include doggy style, or any position that has your partner behind you, side-by-side, and spooning. You should avoid being flat on your back.

Also know this: Sexual frequency and enjoyment drops off sharply in the third trimester, but the desire for noncoital intimacy usually increases. You crave cozy. And of course there are plenty of ways to be intimate with your partner other than intercourse. Cuddle, kiss, and fondle, mutual masturbation and oral sex. Bummer alert: In certain circumstances, your doctor may advise against sex during pregnancy. There are a number of reasons for the O-kill, including placenta previa (a condition in which the placenta partially or wholly blocks the neck of the uterus), ruptured membranes, preterm labor, a shortened cervix, as well as other circumstances that your OB/GYN can discuss with you.

BUT be assured that your baby can't see, feel, or get poked by your partner's penis while you're having sex. So don't worry about that!

FACTOID A recent study found that new moms who are over 34 or have had C-sections can reduce their risk of dangerous blood clots by avoiding hormonal birth control in the first 42 days postpartum. My question is, isn't being postpartum its own form of birth control?!

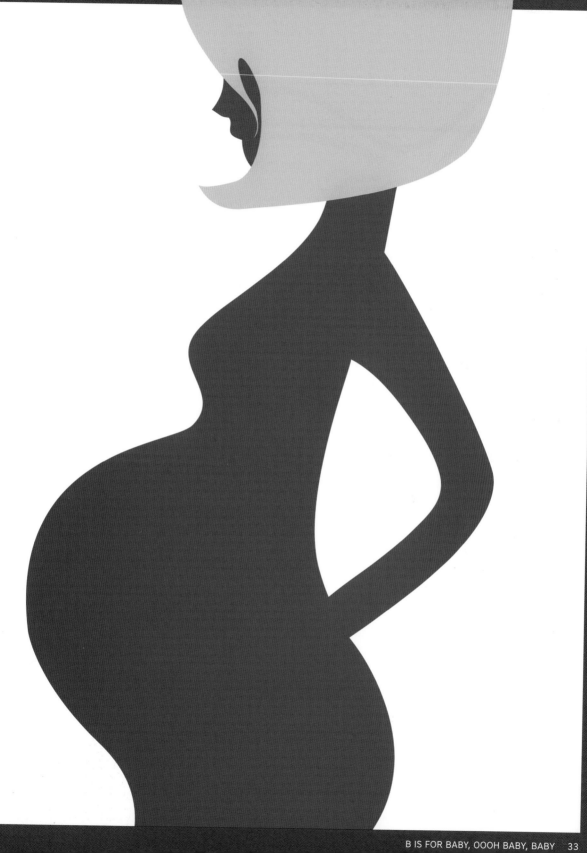

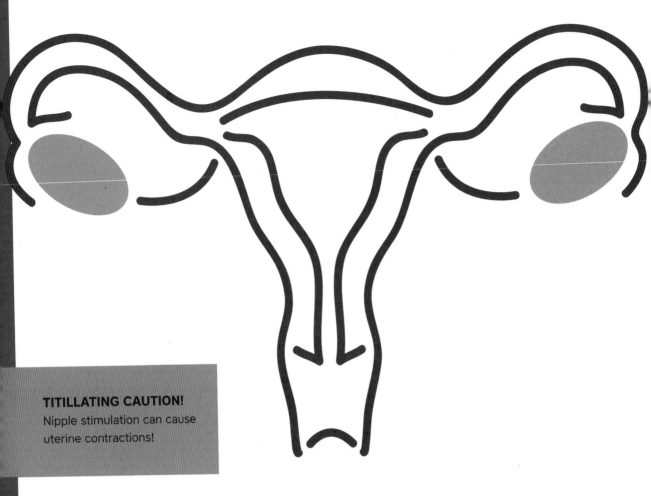

CAN HAVING SEX BRING ON LABOR?

Maybe yes, maybe no. Orgasms involve uterine contractions, and the prostaglandins in ejaculate can also cause your uterine to contract as well as contribute to cervical softening. In low-risk pregnancies, the common thought, therefore, is that having sex is one way to bring on labor.

FACTOID Even if your period has not yet resumed after giving birth or you are breastfeeding, you can become pregnant. Getting pregnant less than six months after giving birth might increase the risk of certain pregnancy problems, such as preterm birth. You should use some type of birth control when you start having sex again.

SEX AFTER BIRTH, OR IS SOMEONE KIDDING ME?

H-e-l-l-o, Libido, are you home? During the postdelivery weeks, everything near the V-zone (or higher up if you've had a C-section) can be mighty sore. Even if you have a sex drive (ha-ha), you're exhausted. As soon as you hit the bed, all you want to do is snore, oh I mean, sleep.

The American Congress of Obstetricians and Gynecologists (ACOG) admits that a six-week hiatus is mostly a random recommendation based on no actual science. But it is true that waiting a little while to resume your sex life after delivery allows time for your cervix to close, postpartum bleeding to stop, and any tears or lacerations to heal. And that doesn't even account for postpartum blues, changes in body image, and other obstacles. (Just reading this is so, so, sexy, right?) All that said, the earliest, exact time at which you can safely start having pain-free intercourse after childbirth is unknown. The truth is, the chances of a problem occurring, like bleeding or infection, are small after about two weeks following birth. If you've had an episiotomy or a tear during birth, however, the site may be sore for a few weeks and you probably should hold off on intercourse until it heals.

Once and if you feel ready to have sex again (some new moms can't wait, while others, not so much!) and your doctor has given you the go-ahead, it's a good idea to use a water-based lubricant and plenty of it. The vagina may be less moist than usual, especially if you are breastfeeding. In fact, some new moms have such notable dryness, caused by a lack of estrogen from nursing, that vaginal estrogen replacement as a cream, a vaginal tablet, or a ring might be a happy option.

Here's what Amy Corbin, blogger for AlphaMom.com, wrote about her six-week, no-sex window:

> While technically my gyno's instructions were simply "nothing in the vagina for six weeks," I chose to interpret it more as "Do not touch me, at all. Do not even think about touching me. Stop looking at me like that." I was so horrified by the state of my body . . . I just couldn't bear the thought of the squishing slapping awkwardness of sex when I didn't recognize the body I now had. What if my boobs leak? What if my stomach dangles?

The surest way to feel good enough to get down again is to discuss your feelings—and the way your body is feeling—honestly and openly with your partner. Whether you want to include in that discussion that you're suddenly feeling like your number-one priority is your amazing baby and not him or her, is up to you. But just know you're not the only woman who ever felt that way.

MORE TIPS You can try urinating every two hours (check the clock) and doing Kegels (pelvic-floor exercises).

I'm worried about giving birth. I've been pretty cool about my pregnancy up until lately, but suddenly I'm realizing that there's a baby that's got to come out and someone is going to have to be there to push it out.

—A Very Pregnant Halle Berry

MY V IS DRIPPING

Well, honey pot, the quantity and quality of vaginal discharge in healthy women varies both individually and during your menstrual cycle. Slight odor and mild irritation can be normal at any time. While pregnant you'll also experience vaginal discharge (called leucorrhea), which will be mucus-like, white or clear, without any other signs and symptoms such as itching, pain, burning or irritation, redness, or bleeding. If you're afraid what you're trickling is actually amniotic fluid (clear, watery vaginal drainage that is continuous and might be copious; most times it's obviously different from the "usual" vaginal discharge experienced day to day, and it may be accompanied by a "popping" sound) or you have an infection, don't hesitate to see your OB.

OMG! WHAT ARE THESE BUMPS?

I'm frequently called by frantic pregnant patients who describe a "cluster of grapes" bulging from their vulvas. Why is it always fruit? We'll discuss that philosophical question another time. For now, more often than not, these are varicose veins of the vulva; in med terms they're known as vulvar varicose veins. Here's what's going on: Now that you're pregnant, the weight of your uterus is pressing down on a major vein, which can slow the return of blood to the heart. The result may be sore, itchy, blue bulges on your legs and vulva. FYI: Hemorrhoids are simply bulging veins in the rectum. In most cases, though you may think they look gross, varicose veins are typically not a problem.

HOW TO DEAL WITH VARICOSE VEINS

Sadly, you can't prevent varicose veins completely. The good news is that you can lessen the chance of getting them or at least limit their severity. Plus, they will usually go away or at least improve after delivery. Meanwhile, here are tips to help relieve swelling and soreness. Bonus: These suggestions may also stop varicose veins from getting worse.

- If you must sit or stand for long periods, be sure to move around from time to time.

- Do not sit with your legs crossed.

- Prop up your legs on your desk, a couch, a chair, or a footstool as often as you can.

- Exercise—walk, swim, or ride an exercise bike.

- Wear support hose.

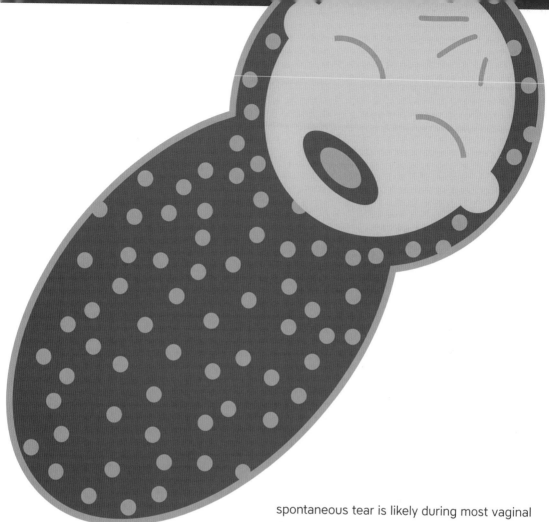

MY GYNO SAID I HAD AN EPISIOTOMY. WHAT EXACTLY IS THAT?

An episiotomy is a cut made by an OB or midwife to your perineum, the space between your vagina and rectum (known colloquially as your "taint," as in it ain't your vagina and it ain't your rectum), in order to make delivery easier. Think: Open wider. And there's no getting around that need for extra space. A

spontaneous tear is likely during most vaginal deliveries, particularly if it's your first. An episiotomy is a way to prevent that tear and control the way that wiggle room is created.

The procedure is pretty common, although not as common as it used to be, as the current thinking is that natural tearing may allow an easier healing period, less chance of tearing extending to the rectum, and perhaps even less pain experienced in sex after delivery. There are a few ways it can be done. One is called a midline, or median, episiotomy, which goes straight from the vaginal opening toward the rectum. Doctors will tell you this type is easiest to perform, repair, and recover from. Also, with this approach, postpartum pain and discomfort during sex is less. The drawback is that there's a higher chance of a tear in the rectum or anal sphincter that can lead to infection and future incontinence. A mediolateral episiotomy is a slightly different version of the procedure in which the incision veers off from the vaginal opening (toward four or eight o'clock if you think of a clock face) as opposed to going straight down toward the rectum (toward six o'clock). This procedure minimizes the chance of sphincter or rectal involvement but has its own downsides: increased blood loss, difficulty with repair, and discomfort postpartum and during sex.

Is there any good news? Yes! Sutures from any repair are absorbable and won't need to be removed by your doc.

FYI Currently, performing an episiotomy as part of a routine delivery is not recommended as it once was, and clinical judgment remains the best guide as to its use. Today it's usually performed only to avoid severe tears and to expedite difficult deliveries.

IT STILL HURTS!

Where? Most likely it's your perineum, the area between your vagina and rectum, that stretches during delivery. This area may feel sore and look swollen and bruised, especially if you had an episiotomy or perineal tear. To ease discomfort and speed healing:

- Apply cold packs or chilled witch-hazel pads to the area.
- Take sitz baths; soaking in a few inches of warm water will bring relief.
- Use a water bottle you can squeeze to soothe the area with a stream of warm water after you urinate.

- Use pain medication.
- Always wipe from front to back after you use the toilet to help prevent a healing episiotomy or tear from getting infected with germs from your rectum.

WHY AM I BLEEDING?

Even though *lochia* sounds like the name of an exotic orchid, it's not so pretty. Lochia refers to the normal shedding of blood and tissue following delivery. For a few days this vaginal discharge is red brown; then it becomes increasingly watery and pinkish brown for a few weeks. Ultimately, the discharge turns yellowish white. Some women continue to pass lochia for six to eight weeks postpartum. Use sanitary pads or panty liners rather than tampons at this time.

I GAVE BIRTH TO A NINE-POUND BABY FIVE WEEKS AGO. MY V IS STILL VERY STRETCHED OUT. WILL IT EVER RETURN TO ITS FORMER TIGHT SELF?

In addition to the size of your baby (big!), there are a number of factors that determine whether or not your vagina will go back to its original size including the kind of operative delivery (forceps or vacuum?), if you've had tears and repairs, your hormone status, the number of children you've had, your overall general health and genetics, and whether you do Kegels regularly. After a vaginal birth, it's expected that the vagina will be larger than it was pre-birth. Though this happens with all vaginal births, you'll probably feel the effects more after a big baby. (Nine pounds [4 kg] definitely qualifies as a big baby!) In this kind of birth, the musculature of the pelvic floor relaxes and loses tone. Not to mention that more tone is lost with each baby you deliver. To this, I say Kegels, Kegels, Kegels!—these exercises will help you get back to normal, or as close as you'll be able to get. There are also several devices available to help deal with vaginal laxity after giving birth. These include vaginal weights and even training trackers that hook up to Bluetooth so that you can monitor your progress (see page 88). Not all are FDA approved, so have a heart-to-heart with your health care professional about possibilities.

See page 114 for info on weight gain during pregnancy.

. . . AND PEEING SO MUCH?

Frequent urination is a common complaint during pregnancy since your kidneys work harder to flush waste products out of your body. In addition, your growing uterus puts pressure on the bladder and your total blood volume increases. Your bladder may be nearly empty but, yes, it still feels like it's full. The weight of your uterus on your bladder may even cause you to leak a little urine when you sneeze or cough. During postpartum, you can experience frequent urination and leakage due to weakened pelvic-floor muscles. It helps to avoid caffeinated drinks since they make you urinate more. But don't be tempted to cut down on other liquids since drinking less could lead to dehydration.

AND WHEN YOU FEEL DISCOURAGED, REMEMBER . . .

A baby is an angel whose wings decrease while his legs increase.

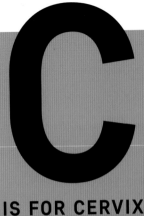

C

IS FOR CERVIX

Pap Smears, HPV, Protection, and
Everything You Need to Know to
Keep Your Lady Flower Safe

Okay, maybe this isn't the sexiest info you'll ever read. It's certainly no Kama Sutra. Still, getting a grip on what's going on in your cervix can be a real lifesaver. Ladies! Please pay attention!

THE PRIMER

Your cervix is made up of several layers of cells. The outer layer is composed of squamous cells. The opening, know as the cervical canal, is made of glandular cells. These two kinds of cells meet in a place called the transformation zone (T-zone). It may sound romantic, but it's really a danger zone because the T-zone is the most common place abnormal cells can be found.

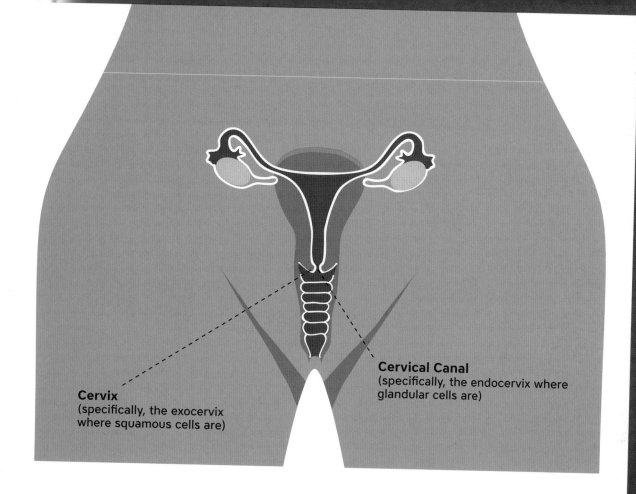

Cervix
(specifically, the exocervix where squamous cells are)

Cervical Canal
(specifically, the endocervix where glandular cells are)

And that's where the Pap test comes in: It screens for cancer of the cervix. Traditionally the Pap test involves collecting a sampling of cells from your cervix using a brush or spatula wielded by your gyno. To get to your cervix, your doc will need to use a speculum (see page 69); the procedure is a little uncomfy, but not painful. The more tense you are, the more uncomfy it will be. I know it's hard to relax when you're bearing it all and propped open with a speculum, but trust me, if you can chill out a bit, things will be much easier for you.

It's a good idea to avoid anything in your vagina a couple of days before your Pap—that means spermicide, lubricant, tampons, and . . . a finger, penis, dildo, etc., as these can disrupt the cells on your cervix and potentially cause an inaccurate reading of the results.

You don't need to get a Pap test before you're 21 years old, and for lots of women, you can get it done every one to three to five years thereafter depending on your risk and age. If you've had a hysterectomy (if performed for a benign or noncancerous condition), Paps aren't necessary unless the cervix is retained. Women over 65 can usually stop having Pap smears.

MY DOCTOR TOLD ME I HAVE HPV. WHAT'S GOING ON?

Unfortunately, these days I'm giving out this same news pretty often. There are more than 100 different strains of HPV and not all of them cause cancer, so it's hard to say exactly what's happening in your case. "Low-risk strains" usually only cause genital warts, which look like little pieces of cauliflower and can appear solo or in groups. "High-risk strains" are linked to cancer of the anus, cervix, vulva, vagina, penis, head, and neck. While close to 80 percent of women are exposed to HPV in their lifetime, the vast majority won't develop cancer.

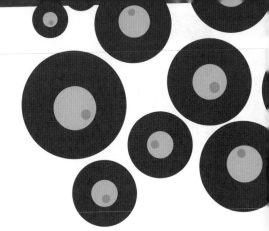

THE LATEST GUIDELINES

- First Pap at 21 years old regardless of whether you have had sex or not

- Ages 21 to 29: Pap every three years. HPV testing not indicated for this age group

- Ages 30 to 65: Pap every three years OR Pap and HPV testing every five years

In truth, many gynos do Pap and HPV co-testing every three years, or even yearly testing, since these are still newish guidelines. A patient may also request testing. If you receive news your Pap test is "abnormal," consult with your health care practitioner about your diagnosis and treatment options.

GOOD NEWS ALERT!

In most cases, the immune system deals with the HPV virus before it causes cancer.

MORE HPV FACTS

- Most women with HPV have no symptoms.

- Most HPV infections are transient and resolve within two years.

- For some women, HPV is persistent and can lead to pre-cancer and then cancer.

- HPV is spread by direct skin-to-skin contact, including sexual intercourse, oral sex, anal sex, and hand-to-genital contact. In fact, newer studies suggest plenty of virgins have HPV, and thus HPV could possibly be transmitted through inanimate objects or surfaces such as medical equipment or sex toys.

- Certain high-risk strains of HPV be tested for alone or in combination with a Pap smear to screen for cervical cancer.

- HPV testing is not recommended for women under 30 years old as this age group's bodies tend to clear virus and cellular abnormalities quickly on their own.

HPV VACCINE FACTS

- There are two available optional vaccines to protect against HPV. Gardasil 9 protects against nine strains of HPV, including multiple high-risk strains, and Cervarix protects against four strains. Both protect against common high-risk strains 16 and 18.

- Neither vaccine will protect against all types of HPV.

- Both are given in two or three doses over a six-month period.

- Vaccines are recommended for girls aged 9 to 26 years. For boys, too!

- Vaccines are best given before a woman is sexually active and is exposed to HPV. However, young women can receive the vaccine even if they have already had sex, had genital warts, have received abnormal Pap test results, or have been infected with HPV.

- If a woman is already infected with one type of HPV, the vaccines will not protect against disease caused by that type.

- Vaccines are not a treatment for current HPV infection.

- The HPV vaccine does not cause HPV.

- Vaccines are not recommended for pregnant women.

- Women who are vaccinated should still have regular Pap tests.

- The most common side effect is soreness in the arm where the shot is given and, rarely, headache, fatigue, nausea, dizziness, and/or fainting.

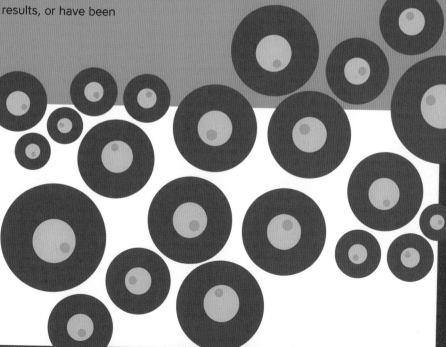

When I told my 13-year-old daughter, Alice, I was taking her to get a vaccine that could help prevent cancer, she was mildly intrigued. "Cool," she allowed, "but I hate shots."

—Claudia Wallis, *Newsweek*

SHOULD EVERYONE GET A COLPOSCOPY?

Hardly! A colposcopy is a test that offers a magnified view of your cervix and V. Your gyno may recommend one if your Pap or HPV test is abnormal, or if you have warts on your cervix, an inflamed cervix (cervicitis), cervical polyps, pain, or bleeding. It's done in the office, takes around 5 to 10 minutes, and is just a little uncomfortable. For at least a day before the test, you should avoid douching (BTW, take this good advice: Never douche!), using tampons, taking vaginal meds, and having sex. It's also a good idea to schedule this test when you're not on a heavy day of menstrual bleeding. Also, avoid anything in your V for a few days after the procedure, and give your doc a buzz immediately if you experience heavy vaginal bleeding, severe lower abdominal pain, fever or chills, or foul discharge. Depending on the results, you may need to be checked more often, or you may need further testing or treatment.

LEEP (LOOP ELECTROSURGICAL EXCISION PROCEDURE) is the most common method for treating significant pre-cancer cells in the cervix, and it is also used to treat the early stage of noninvasive cancer. It's an in-office/outpatient procedure that uses a thin wire loop charged with electric current to remove a cone-shaped area of the cervix, focusing on the small area that contains the abnormality. New healthy cells then regrow. LEEP is reserved for women with high-grade abnormalities since the procedure can potentially cause cervical weakening in subsequent pregnancy.

WHAT IF MY COLPOSCOPY TEST IS WEIRD?

You mean the results showed cells that were abnormal? Well, several treatments are available. Sisters with mild cervical abnormalities, particularly if they're not 30 years old yet, can have their condition monitored with more frequent Paps, HPV tests, and colposcopies as often this abnormality gets better by itself without any treatment. If that's not your case, abnormal cells can be frozen, or removed via laser or surgically.

Newer guidelines suggest we can limit colposcopies even to women over age 24 with Pap test abnormalities because most abnormalities will resolve on their own.

COMPLICATIONS after LEEP or a cone biopsy include bleeding, infection, or weakening of the cervix in future pregnancy. Follow-up testing and treatment depends on results and circumstances.

CERVICAL CANCER

Cervical cancer affects an estimated 12,000 women in the United States each year. About half the cases are in women who have never had a Pap test. The good news: In most cases, cervical cancer can be cured if it's found and treated early. It usually occurs in women older than 40, but anyone can get it. Risk factors include multiple sexual partners, having a male partner who has had multiple sex partners, early age at first intercourse (younger than 18), smoking, family history of cervical cancer, immunosuppression, and in utero exposure to DES (diethylstilbestrol; a medicine used from 1940 to 1971 to prevent miscarriage). Symptoms can include abnormal bleeding or watery vaginal discharge, but it's important to note that many women have no symptoms. A diagnosis is often made after an abnormal Pap leads to a cervical biopsy that confirms the presence of cancer. After diagnosis, the extent of disease is determined with a pelvic exam and various imaging tests of the bladder, rectum, and pelvis. Treatment of cervical cancer depends on how advanced it is but can involve LEEP or cone biopsy, simple or more complex hysterectomy, chemotherapy, and radiation.

There's an excellent chance you can prevent cervical cancer by having regular Pap smears!

D

IS FOR DIAPHRAGM

Plus the Ring, Pill, Patch, Sponge, Condom, Cap, IUD, Abstinence, and Everything You Could Want to Know about Birth Control

Speak to ladies about birth control and you're likely to hear a harangue of horror stories—everything from broken condoms and a surprise trip to Babyville—to cranky caps and free-flying diaphragms. So, let's get real here. Most of us who need, want, and just gotta have birth control (at least for now) want the safest, easiest, most foolproof method in the whole wide universe. Is that too much to ask? Well, maybe. We all have different needs. That's why there's not one simple solution for every fertile femme on the planet. Since we can't just wish upon a star, maybe the best we can hope for is to learn about each method and make a choice based on the facts that fit our lives.

So, let's look at our options . . .

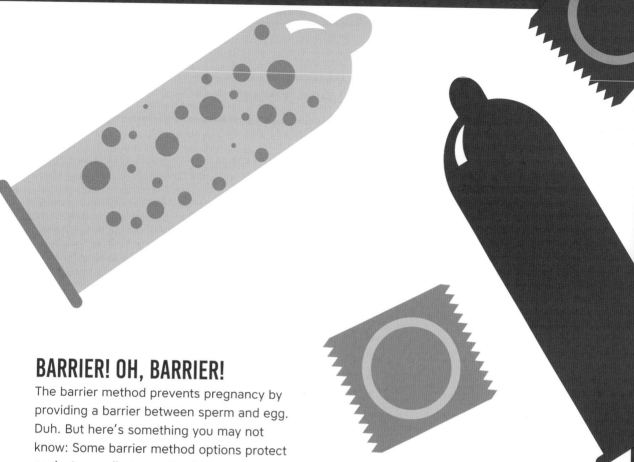

BARRIER! OH, BARRIER!

The barrier method prevents pregnancy by providing a barrier between sperm and egg. Duh. But here's something you may not know: Some barrier method options protect against sexually transmitted diseases, or STDs. The barrier method includes spermicide, diaphragm, cervical cap, condom, female condom, and sponge. What's the good news for those who don't like taking hormones? The barrier method doesn't use any hormones. That's why if you're breastfeeding, barrier methods are a good choice.

Q. What do you get with a corduroy condom?
A. A groovy kind of love!

SPERMICIDE This is a chemical that kills sperm. It comes in different forms: foams, film, creams, jellies, and suppositories. You insert spermicide deep into your vagina just before having sexual intercourse. Spermicides provide some pregnancy protection when used alone, but they work much better when combined with a condom, diaphragm, or cervical cap. FYI: Read directions carefully and don't douche! As discussed in chapter P, you should never douche, and when it comes to sex, douching after sex will not prevent pregnancy and it may predispose you to infection.

Noise alert! One patient described sex with a female condom as sounding like a pack of M&M's ripping open in a movie theater.

—Dr. Dweck

DIAPHRAGM Seen any UFOs between your legs? A diaphragm is a round and dome-shaped reusable latex insert with a firm but flexible rim. It is placed inside your vagina before sexual intercourse to cover your cervix (the opening to the uterus) so that sperm can't enter. A diaphragm should be used with spermicidal cream or jelly.

Some men are sponge-worthy, and some men are just not sponge-worthy.
—Elaine on *Seinfeld*

CONDOMS Thin barriers made of latex, plastic, or natural membranes. They look like long, thin, deflated balloons. There are both male and female condoms. The male condom fits over a man's penis. The female condom fits inside a woman's vagina. Both male and female condoms work by preventing sperm from entering the vagina and reaching an egg.

SPONGE A disc-shaped birth control device made of soft foam coated with spermicide. It's inserted vaginally to cover your cervix and can be worn for up to 30 hours and put in place up to 24 hours before sex. One sponge allows for lots of acts of intercourse in a 24-hour period (yay!), but there's a 16 to 30 percent failure rate (boo!). DON'T use the sponge during your period, if you're less than six weeks postpartum, or you have had toxic shock syndrome (TSS) in the past.

CERVICAL CAP A small latex cup that you insert into your vagina before sexual intercourse. The cervical cap, which needs to be fitted by a health professional, slips snugly over your cervix. It's similar to a diaphragm in that it blocks the cervix so sperm can't enter the uterus and it must be used with spermicidal cream or jelly. It is, however, smaller than the diaphragm.

FACTOID Twenty-nine percent of men and 32 percent of women report knowing "little or nothing about condoms."

HOW TO USE YOUR DIAPHRAGM

You can get a diaphragm through your doctor, who can teach you how to use it. If you skipped the lesson, forgot, or just want to know what to anticipate, here's a step-by-step guide:

1. Wash your hands with soap and water.
2. Inspect the diaphragm for holes.
3. Put approximately one tablespoon of spermicidal cream or jelly in the cup and around the rim.
4. Sit, squat, lie down, or stand with one foot up on a chair and get comfortable.
5. Separate the lips of the vagina with one hand, and with the other hand, pinch the rim of the diaphragm to fold it in half and then insert it into the vagina; push it up as far as it will go; the firm part of the rim should be felt behind your pubic bone, comfortably against the cervix (see page 41 for a diagram).
6. Check to see whether your cervix is covered by reaching inside—the cervix feels firm like the tip of your nose.
7. A diaphragm can be inserted up to 6 hours prior to sex and must be left in for at least 6 but no more than 24 hours afterward. Do not remove the diaphragm if you have sex more than once within 6 hours; just insert more spermicide.
8. Spermicidal jelly should be applied no more than 2 hours prior to sex and with each sex act, no matter how close in time.
9. To remove your diaphragm, wash hands with soap and water, hook a finger over the rim to break the suction, then pull the diaphragm down and out.
10. Upon removing the diaphragm, wash with warm soap and water and store in its case.
11. Avoid oil-based lubricants or talc.
12. Avoid use if you have a latex allergy or sensitivity to spermicides.

Use your diaphragm at every conceivable chance.

Q. What's a diaphragm?
A. A trampoline for dickheads.

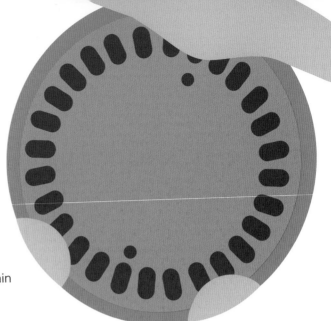

HORMONES! HELP!

Hormonal methods of birth control include the pill, the ring, the patch, the shot, and the implant. In a nutshell, the combination pill, patch, and ring prevent ovulation. They contain synthetic estrogen and progestin (that's the combo part), which stabilize hormone levels and prevent the midcycle estrogen surge. As a result, the pituitary gland (a gland in the brain that regulates ovulation, among other things) does not release follicle stimulating hormone (FSH) and luteinizing hormone (LH), the typical signals to the ovaries to release a mature egg, and this is how ovulation is suppressed.

The progestin hormone in the pill also supports the uterine lining to prevent breakthrough bleeding. Synthetic progestin may also

- stop the pituitary gland from producing LH in order to prevent ovulation;

- make the uterine lining inhospitable to a fertilized egg;

- limit sperm's ability to fertilize the egg; and

- thicken the cervical mucus to hinder sperm movement.

There are progesterone-only methods of hormonal birth control, and they can be administered through a shot, patch, implant, the "mini" pill, and even IUDs that contain progesterone. These methods may but don't always suppress ovulation.

ORAL CONTRACEPTION, AKA THE PILL When it comes to the pill, there are many brands and formulas available containing different levels of estrogen and progestin. Some pills allow for a monthly cycle, while others will give a period every three months or not at all. Talk to your doctor about which pill might be the best one for you. Also discuss its side effects. While you're at it, bring up the possibility of taking the mini pill, which contains only progesterone and no estrogen and is therefore ideal for women who smoke, are over 35, or are breastfeeding, though it is a smidge less reliable than the combination pill. FYI: Fertility returns as soon as you stop taking any kind of birth control pill—like the next day.

A PRESCRIPTION is required for all of these methods, and none of them protect against STDs.

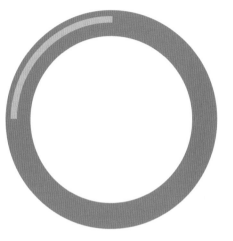

My best birth control these days is just to leave the lights on.

—Joan Rivers

VAGINAL RING (NuvaRing) This is a flexible plastic ring, easily inserted vaginally, that releases both estrogen and progestin. It's placed for 21 days and then is removed for 7 days, at which time you'll get your period. If you prefer, the ring can be used continuously and changed every three weeks so that you don't menstruate at all. Follow the instructions carefully.

PATCH (Ortho Evra) If you choose the contraceptive patch, you'll be wearing pregnancy-preventing hormones instead of swallowing them in pill form. Made of plastic, the size of a small matchbook, and designed to stick to your skin, the contraceptive patch works by releasing hormones that are absorbed through your skin and then go directly into your bloodstream. Your job is to replace it with a new patch every week. Failure rate is higher for woman over 198 pounds. Also, a blood clot may be more likely to develop in women on the patch than on the pill.

IMPLANT (Nexplanon) This is a progestin-only itty-bitty "rod" that is inserted under the skin in the upper arm by your health care provider. It works for up to three years and is easily reversible with removal. A big advantage is that you don't have to remember it every day, or even every month. Bonus: You can be sexually spontaneous. Quickie, anyone?

THE SHOT (Depo-Provera) This is an every-three-months injection of progestin (DPMA). One disadvantage: A lot of women gain weight with the shot.

FROM THE JUST-DO-SOMETHING FILES As many as half of the pregnancies in the United States are unplanned!

IUD The IUD is a small, T-shaped piece of flexible plastic that fits inside your uterus to prevent pregnancy. There are two types of IUDs: copper and progestin (a hormone found in birth control pills). The copper IUD can last ten years and works by interfering with the sperm's ability to reach the egg. The progestin IUD can last three or five years depending on the type and works predominantly by thickening cervical mucus and thinning the uterine lining.

MORNING-AFTER PILL (Oops!) Alert! This is not a contraceptive for regular use. Instead, it's a treatment to prevent pregnancy after unprotected sex or a mishap with the barrier method (a broken condom, for example). It can be bought over the counter if you are 18 years or older. Take it as soon as possible. Studies show the morning-after pill is most effective if taken within five days of having unprotected sex. This is not an abortion pill. It is postcoital contraception and prevents pregnancy from occurring about 75 percent of the time when taken correctly.

FYI Before deciding on any method of birth control, speak with your doctor and talk it over with your partner. Go over the risks of pregnancy involved (they all have some—from less than 1 percent to much higher), side effects (if any), and directions.

WHAT DOESN'T PROTECT YOU FROM PREGNANCY?

DOUCHING Squirting water or any other liquid into the vagina after sex does not kill sperm or prevent pregnancy.

PLASTIC WRAP INSTEAD OF A CONDOM Plastic wrap or a plastic bag can tear and let sperm escape.

URINATING RIGHT AFTER SEX Urine does not pass through the vagina, so it does not get rid of the sperm.

HAVING SEX FOR THE FIRST TIME You can get pregnant even if you have never had sex before.

A SPECIAL POSITION No matter which way you're standing, sitting, kneeling, or whatever, if his penis enters—or comes close to—your vagina, sister, you can get knocked up.

IF YOU'RE SURE YOU DON'T WANT A BABY

Tubal ligation (having your "tubes tied") is a surgical procedure that cuts, seals, or blocks the fallopian tubes to prevent pregnancy. There is no hormonal change. This is typically an outpatient procedure done in a minimally invasive way; it can also be done at the time of cesarean section. Anesthesia is required. Failure rate is less than 1 percent. However, the risk of ectopic pregnancy (nonviable pregnancy found outside the uterus usually in the fallopian tube) is rare but possible. The procedure is considered permanent, and reversal is not straightforward.

Tubal occlusion procedures include Essure. This allows for a tiny coil to be placed into the fallopian tubes through a telescope (hysteroscope) that is placed into the vagina and then into the cervix and uterus. Scar tissue then develops around the coil, causing the tubes to become sealed shut. This outpatient procedure requires at least local anesthesia. A confirmatory X-ray type test called an HSG (hysterosalpingogram) is done three months later to confirm the tubes are fully blocked. As many as 15 percent of women will need to have the procedure repeated.

Vasectomy is a surgical sterilization procedure for guys that cuts or blocks the vas deferens, the tubes that carry sperm from the testes. It is an office procedure done under local anesthesia. It takes up to three months to be effective. The failure rate is less than 1 percent.

Birth control that really works? Every night before we go to bed we spend an hour with our kids.

—Roseanne Barr

ARE THERE OTHER OPTIONS?

Well, there's abstinence, which means choosing to abstain from sexual intercourse, while you still can engage in other sexual activities. Some people choose to abstain from all sexual activity. When practiced, abstinence is the only 100 percent fail-proof way to prevent pregnancy. But it's not much fun.

Planned abstinence means trying to predict the time of the month when fertility is highest and avoiding sex at that time. Here's how:

Rhythm or calendar method uses the first day of your last period to determine your most fertile time. Ladies with a 28- to 30-day cycle (from day 1 of bleeding to day 1 of bleeding in next cycle) should avoid sex from days 10 to 19. This method is not recommended if you have irregular cycles or you're nursing.

Basal body temperature method relies on the fact that your morning temperature (taken before you get out of bed) will rise slightly, half a degree Fahrenheit, after ovulation. Thus, sex should be avoided midcycle, on or around ovulation, to prevent pregnancy. In a 28-day cycle with peak temperature on day 14, avoid sex approximately on days 10 through 18. Sex from day 1 until temperature elevation should be safe. This may not work if you are nursing or nearing menopause.

Cervical mucus is typically more watery and heavier when you're ovulating. To prevent pregnancy, you should avoid sex when watery cervical mucus first appears until three or four days after the heaviest day of mucus.

Withdrawal, or coitus interruptus, means your man pulls his penis from your vagina before he ejaculates. This won't work if he withdraws too late or if sperm are released before the big explosion.

Breastfeeding delays the return of ovulation. That's why it can be somewhat effective in preventing pregnancy, particularly in those who nurse exclusively for the first six months and don't menstruate. However, as we learned in the B chapter, you can still get pregnant at this time, as you don't know when ovulation will start again prior to the return of your first period—it's just less likely.

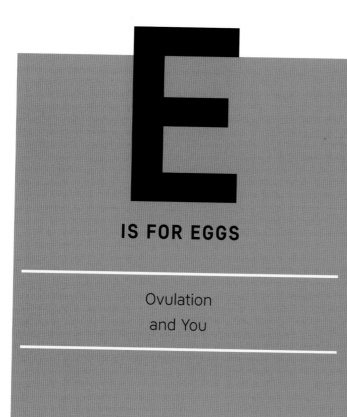

E

IS FOR EGGS

Ovulation
and You

LESSON 101: OVULATION (OR HORMONAL CYCLE/LH SURGE)

What is ovulation, exactly? Well, it's simply the monthly release of your egg from your ovary. In an average 28-day menstrual cycle, ovulation occurs about 14 days after the first day of your last period. (FYI: "Day 1" always means the first day of your period.) It's like this: Each month an egg matures in a menstruating woman's ovary. The egg is surrounded by a sac called a follicle. The cells of the follicle first produce the hormone estrogen. This triggers a surge of LH (luteinizing hormone) from the pituitary gland in the brain, and the egg is then released. The follicle cells then begin to produce progesterone

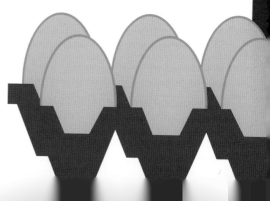

It is a well-documented fact that guys will not ask for directions. This is a biological thing. This is why it takes several million sperm cells . . . to locate a female egg, despite the fact that the egg is, relative to them, the size of Wisconsin.

—Dave Barry

as well as estrogen. This prepares the uterine lining for pregnancy if fertilization occurs. If pregnancy does not occur (and depending on where you're at, that's good or bad news), the egg degenerates and the thickened uterine lining sheds—and then you get your period, which is the shedding of that lining.

If you want to get pregnant, you should try to have sex every other day for about a week around the time of ovulation—horny or not. To prevent pregnancy, use contraception or avoid sex when you are ovulating.

HOW CAN I TELL WHEN OR EVEN IF I'M OVULATING?

You can do it. Trust me. Chart your cycle on a calendar for a few months. If you have a regular 28-day cycle, with day 1 being the first day of your menses, you will typically ovulate on or around day 14. If you have a shorter or longer cycle, you can count backward 14 days from the first day of your period and that will usually be ovulation day. There are a few ways to keep track of your cycle.

TRACK YOUR SYMPTOMS

Most of us will experience one or more of these:

- A twinge of discomfort when we ovulate.

- Breast soreness.

- Just before ovulation, more cervical mucus is produced and it becomes clear, slippery, and stretchy. Think raw egg white.

- Increase in horniness.

FACTOID Whaaaa? If you're ovulating, it turns out a guy's nose knows it. The olfactory signal automatically boosts his testosterone making him primed for a romp in the sheets, reports a study from Florida State University and reported in the journal *Psychological Science*.

MONITOR YOUR BASAL TEMPERATURE

Your basal temperature (the lowest temperature your body attains during rest or sleep) increases about one-half degree after ovulation. To do this, take your temperature first thing in the morning at the same time every day before you even get out of bed. Chart your temperature on a graph that also shows your menstrual cycle. You should see a pattern of slight temperature increase approximately 24 to 48 hours after you ovulate. In subsequent months, you can then predict when you will ovulate.

USE AN OVULATION PREDICTOR KIT OR A FERTILITY MONITOR

You can get these kits over-the-counter at most drugstores. They're urine tests that measure your LH, which is a hormone produced by the pituitary gland in your brain. The LH surge predicts ovulation within approximately 24 hours.

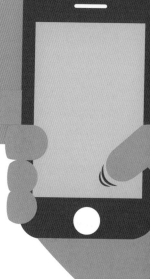

THERE'S AN APP FOR THAT!

Hey, even better: Use an app! There are apps for everything from monitoring your period and all-important mucus, to charting your fertile times of the month, even prompting when you should have intercourse to boost your chances of getting pregnant.

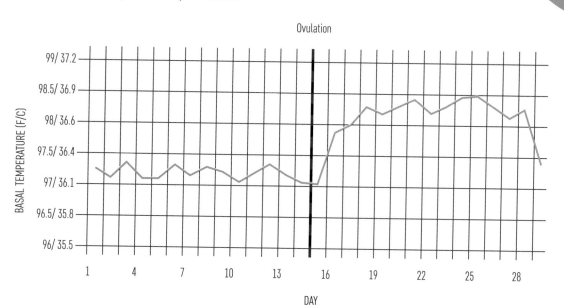

If it's so hard to get pregnant, how do you account for the number of crying children on planes?

—Samantha on *Sex and the City*

I ALWAYS KNOW WHEN I'M OVULATING BECAUSE IT, LIKE, KILLS!

Welcome to the world of Mittelschmerz. Yeah, it sounds like a German opera but it literally means "middle pain," and it's the word for the discomfort felt when you're ovulating. For some of us, it's a mild twinge or cramp in the lower belly or back. But for some ladies, ovulation is an intense pain. The ache can alternate sides, and, like clockwork, it happens every month during the midcycle. It can last minutes or hours and usually feels sharp and crampy. Bloating and discomfort can occasionally last for 24 to 48 hours. You can treat Mittelschmerz with ibuprofen a day before you're expecting the discomfort and by using a heating pad when pain strikes. Birth control pills are also a common treatment. Why? Because they prevent ovulation. If your Mittelschmerz symptoms last longer than two or three days, tell your doctor about it since there might be another reason why you're in pain.

WE'VE BEEN TRYING FOR WELL OVER A YEAR AND HAVEN'T GOTTEN PREGNANT. WHAT'S UP WITH THAT?

Well, that depends. Here's the math: We're born with about 1 to 2 million eggs. By puberty about 300,000 to 400,000 are still there. Of these, about 300 to 400 will be ovulated during a woman's reproductive lifetime. You never produce new eggs—ever. (Men, on the other hand, produce sperm continuously throughout most of their lives.) Eggs degenerate during pregnancy, with the use of birth control pills, and just naturally as we age, until menopause when they're all gone.

REALLY? Ovulating women have more accurate gaydar than the rest of us, according to a study in the journal *Psychological Science*. This is at least partly because they are better able to subconsciously pick up on mating cues from males. Hmmmmmm . . .

OVARIAN RESERVE

This term refers to the number and quality of your eggs and thus to your ability to get pregnant. Since lots of modern ladies choose to delay childbearing for various reasons, including furthering their careers and education, ovarian reserve and the testing for it are more relevant than ever before. Sadly, the truth is that the decline in ovarian reserve is irreversible. It's affected by:

- **AGE** Possibly as young as 32, definitely by 35, and even more so by 40

- **ENVIRONMENTAL FACTORS** such as smoking, or a history of chemotherapy or radiation

- **GENETICS** Family history of early menopause and personal history of having had ovarian surgery such as ovarian cyst removal or ovary removal

TESTING

Having your ovarian reserve tested typically involves blood testing for the hormones FSH and estradiol on day 2 of your menstrual cycle. An anti-mullerian hormone (AMH) test can be done at any time of your cycle. Traditionally, if a day-2 FSH comes back at a value over 12 and/ or a random-day AMH test comes back with a value less than 1, that might suggest diminished ovarian reserve and a tendency toward fertility challenges. But don't jump to conclusions too quickly! Values vary by lab, so be sure to have an in-depth discussion with your doctor about the results. And remember, ovarian reserve isn't the only piece of the puzzle, and more advanced testing is available.

FACTOID Trouble getting pregnant? You're not alone. According to the CDC (Centers for Disease Control and Prevention), the number of American women aged 15 to 44 who have ever used infertility services is 7.3 million.

CAN IT BE POSSIBLE THAT I'VE NEVER OVULATED EVEN THOUGH I SOMETIMES GET MY PERIOD?

Yup. Polycystic ovary syndrome (PCOS) is a condition in which ovulation doesn't occur or occurs infrequently due to an imbalance in hormones. Sisters with PCOS produce an excess amount of male hormones called androgens. These women usually have irregular menstrual bleeding or no menses at all and often have trouble getting pregnant. Some have acne and unwanted hair growth in typically male places like the upper lip and chin, between their breasts, on the lower part of the abdomen, and on the inner thighs. Many with PCOS produce too much insulin, and that which is produced doesn't work well. This results in obesity and difficulty losing and maintaining weight. The risk of diabetes, uterine cancer, high blood pressure, and heart disease is higher than in women who don't have PCOS. There are treatments, though. They include diet (healthier with calorie restriction for weight loss), exercise, hair removal, oral anti-diabetic medications, and birth control pills. Fertility treatment is often needed to assist with pregnancy.

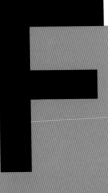

F

IS FOR FUNGUS

And Other Infections That
Make Us Feel Funky

Oh why oh why is the word "fun" in the word *fungus*? Pshht. The irony! I admit, fungus is not the most tasteful teatime conversation, but let's just deal and get it over with. BTW: That's good advice if you have a vaginal yeast infection.

Here's the scoop: A small amount of clear or cloudy white fluid passing each day from your V is totally normal. Think of this discharge as a lovely moisturizer because, darling, that's what it is. It keeps your lady flower's tissue moist and healthy. And don't fret over a small diff in the amount or color because it usually changes throughout your menstrual cycle and can vary from girlfriend to girlfriend.

In response to calls for sexual equality, Pillsbury recently added a new Pillsbury Dough Girl. Unfortunately, she missed her first day of work because she had a yeast infection. Ha-ha-ha.

As with almost all things related to the body, if you ask the Internet about something you're experiencing, you'll likely come up with some really crazy and utterly incorrect answers. When it comes to lady fluids, there is a lot of discussion online shaming anyone who has any secretion on their panties—ever. Let me reassure you, some discharge on some, or even all, days is the norm for some women. Certainly, increased amounts midcycle with ovulation is normal! Did you hear me? NORMAL! Anyway, I digress; your V contains lots of organisms including yeast and bacteria. But sometimes conditions go awry. Let's take a quick peek at some things that can happen.

YEAST Vaginal yeast infections are caused by a friend you don't want to see, the fungus called *Candida*. It's totally common and can visit sisters of any age. The usual symptom is an itchy vulva and vagina. You might also have a thick, white clumpy vaginal discharge resembling cottage cheese, plus other symptoms like pain or burning while urinating, vulvar soreness or irritation, discomfort during sex, and a red, swollen vulva and vagina. You raise your risk for getting a yeast infection with antibiotic use, hormonal contraceptives, devices like the sponge or diaphragm, constantly

wearing panty liners or panty hose, and sitting around in your wet swimsuit or workout clothes. Yeast infections are more common if you have a weakened immune system from infection such as HIV or certain medications like steroids or chemotherapy, or if you're pregnant or have diabetes (especially if sugar levels aren't controlled). Even though yeast infections are not an STD, they can happen more frequently when you're having sex, especially oral.

Treatment of yeast infections includes either an oral pill or a topical vaginal treatment with cream or suppository. If it's a simple yeast infection, it will probably go away in a few days with treatment. If you get recurrent infections (more than four a year), you might need treatments repeated. Since vaginal yeast infections are rarely passed from one partner to another, treatment for your sex partner is generally not recommended. But there are exceptions, as when your partner has symptoms (which in men can be redness, a rash, and the same kind of itching and burning we ladies endure).

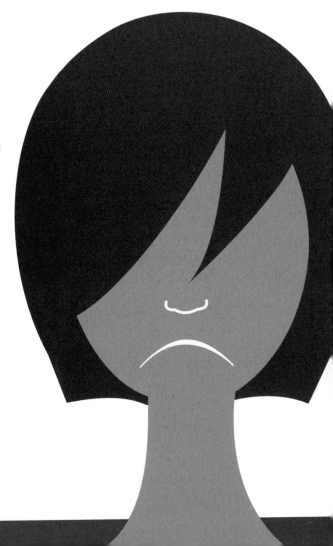

FYI Lots of ladies self-treat with OTC (over-the-counter) medication when they think it's a yeast infection. Sometimes they're mistaken, and this can make the right diagnosis more challenging for a gyno, because the wrong treatment can cause further irritation. It's a vicious cycle, frustrating for you—and your doc.

VAGINITIS Uh . . . did you forget that tampon? I'm only asking because a vaginal infection is often the body's reaction to an imbalance in the usual V organisms commonly caused by something foreign inside it. You won't believe how many times women come into my office because of a forgotten tampon—and believe me, you can smell it a mile away or, more likely, from the waiting room. Excuse my candor, but it happens. If you've experienced it, you've likely felt pretty silly, but at least you know now that you're not alone. It could also be a misplaced condom causing symptoms. Other vaginitis triggers are spermicide containing nonoxynol-9 (check labels carefully) or heavily fragrant soap or body wash, or hormonal changes like menopause or pregnancy. Hey, if you've got itching of the vulva, vagina or labia, redness, burning, soreness or swelling of the vulvar skin, a stinky odor, foamy or green/yellow or bloody discharge, pain with sex or urination, abdominal or pelvic pain, think vaginitis and then see your gyno ASAP.

BACTERIAL VAGINOSIS (BV) Got BV? Well, it's hard to miss. You'll get the hint because there will be a noticeable increase in discharge (thin and gray), along with a strong fishy odor. You might also be itchy down there and bleed after sex. What's the cause for all this V havoc? Simply an imbalance in bacteria types that can develop thanks to multiple or new sexual partners, douching and/or cigarette smoking, or just because . . . who knows? Sometimes we don't! Even though BV is not thought to be an STD, it is more common when you're having sex. BV itself is not harmful, but it can increase the risk of HIV infection and transmission and other STDs, preterm delivery in pregnant women, and postsurgical infection. Your gyno can make a diagnosis and prescribe the proper treatment that will mean taking antibiotics either orally or intra-vaginally. Note: BV can happen again and again, and if that's the case, you'll need more frequent or longer rounds of antibiotics. A good way to avoid all this V drama is to use condoms.

Sometimes, if a case of BV is really tough to get rid of, I'll prescribe boric acid vaginal suppositories (yes, the stuff that kills roaches!) to keep the vaginal pH in balance and prevent recurrent or chronic BV. Boric acid supplements are usually made in special compounding pharmacies, not your typical drugstore chain. There are also OTC products that claim to keep the vaginal pH in line such as probiotics.

USE IT OR LOSE IT Regular sexual activity maintains a healthy, juicy, lovely lady flower, so long as you're practicing good hygiene and using lube if you experience dryness. If you have a lot of sex with a partner or through masturbation, your V will stay elastic and pliable. Go for it!

ATROPHIC VAGINITIS Add this condition to the list titled "Bummers of Getting Older." You get atrophic vaginitis when you stop producing estrogen and your poor, tired lady flower loses her blossom and elasticity and gets thin and delicate and, well, dries up. Hold on! It's not always menopause doing the damage. It could be lactation, a postpartum period, or during administration of anti-estrogenic drugs. And the change in your V doesn't happen overnight. Still, you'll notice it. There might be inflammation, thinning of the vaginal and lower urinary tract tissue, shortening and narrowing of the V canal with loss of stretching ease and less juice. Plus, you can be more susceptible to trauma. In other words, you might bleed even during a routine pelvic exam or Pap test. As if that's not enough, thinning tissue can often cause itching, burning, infection, painful sex, bleeding, and urinary discomfort and frequency. Your gyno can give you the bad news. Any good news? Yes! Your symptoms can be managed if you regularly use a vaginal moisturizer in much the same way you use body lotion every day. Popular brands are Replens and Luvena. My favorite is Sexcellence, a compounded vaginal moisturizer containing hyaluronic acid, vitamin E and aloe. Meanwhile, lubricants can be used on demand for sex. Popular choices are K-Y Jelly, Astroglide, SYLK, and Überlube.

PREADOLESCENT VAGINITIS

This condition can result from infection, congenital abnormality, trauma and sexual abuse, dermatologic conditions, foreign body (toilet paper is the most common), and pinworm to name a few. Because pre-pubertal hypo-estrogenic tissues are thin and delicate, they're more susceptible to local irritants, foreign bodies, and infection. Moms, be open with your daughters about their bodies, and that will go a long way to keeping them healthy. If you have an open dialogue with them, they will be more comfortable with their bodies and more likely to get to the doc quick if they need treatment.

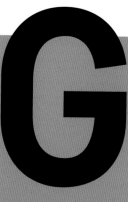

G

IS FOR GYNO

A Guide to Wellness Visits and
Getting Down with Your Gyno

It's too bad you probably don't think there's anything funny about going to the gyno. If you're like most ladies, you have like a million, no, make that a gazillion, reasons not to see your gynecologist: You might be embarrassed because you have an STD or just think you have one (an excellent reason to be on the examining table!). Maybe you haven't had anything abnormal going on down there, so you don't feel like making the trip. Or you could just be shy, and showing your lady flower to a doctor is the last thing in the world you want to do. Perhaps you have a ton of anxiety wrapped up with what could go wrong, and you'd rather bring Voldemort home as your date than get into the stirrups. Okay, that's extreme but you get my point—you have your

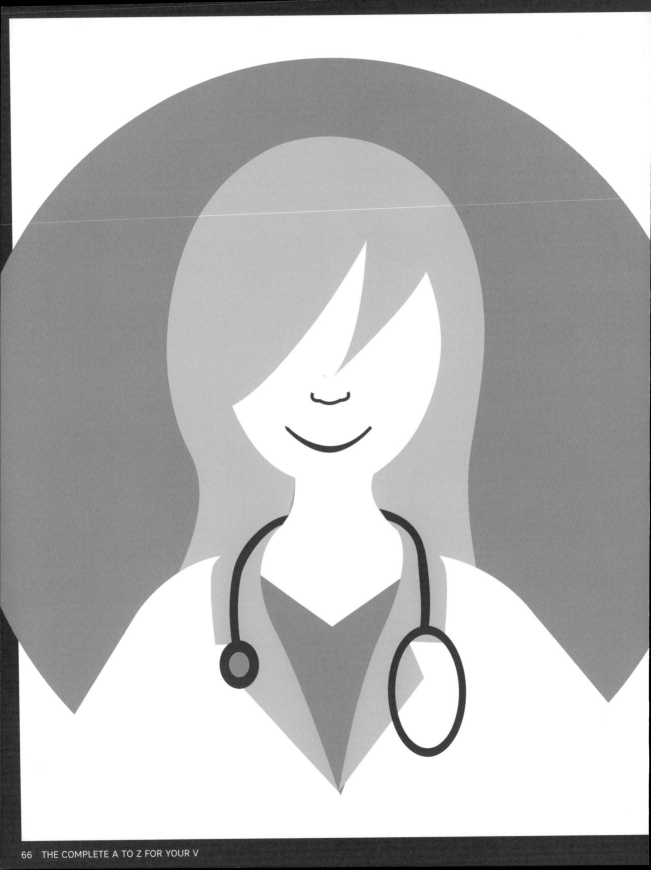

reasons. Whatever they are, girl, get over them! Keeping your lady flower in good health is one of the best things you can do for yourself, and there's no reason on earth that trumps your own health and well-being.

Q. What's the difference between a genealogist and a gynecologist?
A. A genealogist looks up your family tree. A gynecologist looks up your family bush!

MY GYNECOLOGIST ASKED ME A MILLION QUESTIONS BEFORE I EVEN SPREAD MY LEGS. IS THIS NORMAL OR IS SHE JUST BEING NOSY?

Sounds like you have a good gynecologist; don't hold back. Blab on! The more information physicians have, the better they can treat their patients.

When you go to a gyno for the first time, here's what you should be asked:

- The reason for your visit (you should be asked this even if it's not your first visit to that doc), your age, and your obstetrical history, which includes info about prior pregnancies (whether you have had vaginal or cesarean deliveries, miscarriages, abortions, any complications or unique circumstances that are pertinent to each). You should also be questioned about your menstrual history (age at first menses or menopause, cycle regularity, flow amount and length, issues with cramps or abnormal bleeding, issues with hot flashes or night sweats, and whether you use tampons or pads, including any problems inserting tampons). Stay put; we're not done yet . . .

- You should also be asked about results of prior Pap tests and treatments for any abnormalities.

- Have you had prior or frequent infections or STDs, ovarian cysts, uterine fibroids, polyps, endometriosis, polycystic ovaries, or exposure to DES (diethylstilbestrol, a synthetic form of estrogen used in the middle of the twentieth century)?

- Any trouble with urinating or moving your bowels? And we're still not done . . .

- On to your sexual history: Are you currently having sex and, if so, with men, women, or both? Do you have multiple partners? What do you use for contraception (past and present)? Is sex painful? Do you suffer from vaginal dryness? Do you have libido or orgasm issues?

- Also, what medications do you take including prescription meds, OTC meds, vitamins, or supplements? Do you have allergies to any medications?

- Then there's your general medical history: Do you have any current or past issues with the heart, lungs, thyroid, kidney, liver; bleeding or clotting problems; psychiatric problems; or any prior hospitalizations and, if so, for what? Have you had surgery before? Let's take a breather . . . Okay, onward!

> *A male gynecologist is like an auto mechanic who has never owned a car.*
>
> —Carrie P. Snow, Comedian

- Lifestyle habits: Do you smoke and, if so, how much? Do you drink alcohol and, if so, how much? Do you use drugs? Are you married, single, partnered, divorced, or widowed? Are you the victim of any abuse? Are you a student, or do you work and, if so, what do you do? Do you exercise regularly?

- Your doctor will also want to know about your family history, specifically whether there are female cancers in the family (parents, siblings, grandparents). For example, this includes positive genetic testing for the BRCA gene (finding changes in these genes, called BRCA1 and BRCA2, can help determine your chance of developing breast cancer and ovarian cancers). Similarly, your gyno will want to know about immediate relatives with blood clots or heart disease.

Now that your practitioner has a handle on your medical history and concerns, it's time for the exam.

"What about a combination gynecologist and bikini waxer?"
"That is literally a one-stop pussy shop."
—Abbi and Ilana
talking on *Broad City*

WHAT SHOULD A GOOD ANNUAL EXAM BE LIKE?

Typically, a nurse or medical assistant will take your weight (in my office, women will remove belts, shoes, clothes, and even jewelry to be weighed. Wedding rings? Yes!), blood pressure, pulse, and temperature. Your doc or nurse-practitioner may also check your skin for rashes, discoloration, and temperature; your neck for enlarged glands; and your thyroid gland for nodules or enlargement. Also, a breast exam is typically done first in the sitting position then lying down checking for symmetry, pain, lumps, skin changes, nipple discharge, and armpit lumps. Your gyno should also feel your abdomen for pain, masses, or enlarged organs.

I NEVER KNOW WHAT MY DOCTOR IS DOING DOWN THERE.

You're lying down on the exam table with your feet in stirrups, feeling totally exposed and vulnerable. Hello, cowgirl! You're getting a pelvic exam. I've done several thousand of them, so let me tell you about it: First your external V is inspected carefully, which includes inspection of the pubic hair distribution, skin, labia (minora and majora), clitoris, urethral opening, and the various glands, hymen or hymeneal remnants (such as subtle scarring or changes in contour that formed when the hymen broke), and anus.

Now for the "fun" part: A speculum is gently (note the adverb!) inserted into your vajayjay to check out your vaginal walls and cervix and may take swabs for infection and, if needed, a Pap test. Next, a bimanual exam is done in which your gyno inserts one or two fingers of one hand vaginally to palpate and elevate your pelvic organs while using the other hand to sweep your abdominal organs downward in order to evaluate the cervix, uterus, and ovaries and check for size, pain, mobility, and consistency. Had enough? Maybe not. A rectal exam is occasionally done to feel the back of the uterus and ovaries and to check for rectal irregularities, blood in the stool, and pelvic masses in those who are too young to tolerate a vaginal exam.

POSSIBLE TESTS

Certain tests may be taken including a Pap test with or without an HPV test, cultures for infection, and blood and urine tests. In addition, your gyno may order or perform a pelvic ultrasound, a mammogram and ultrasound of the breasts, and a bone density test, and/or recommend immunizations or consults with other docs.

Then she took out a speculum the size of a milkshake machine.

—Tina Fey, *Bossypants*

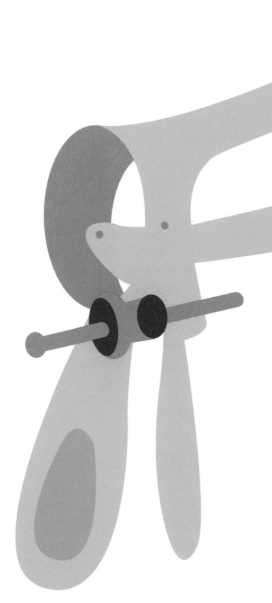

HEY, WHAT'S WITH THAT TOTALLY SCARY SPECULUM?

Okay, okay, sure I get it, but it can't be helped. Gynecologists need to use a speculum to look inside your vagina and see your cervix clearly. Squeamish alert: Ready? There are a wide variety of vaginal specula (metal or plastic, narrow or wide, long or pediatric size) that can be used by a gynecologist to perform an examination. Most of these devices have two blades (not at all sharp—that's just what you call that shape) and a handle. They look like duck bills. Once the blades are clicked into place, the handle can be locked by fastening a screw. It helps to breathe deeply if you're feeling anxious. Who wouldn't be?

HOW OFTEN SHOULD I HAVE A WELLNESS VISIT?

I want to talk about something that's going around lately that really gets plenty of gynos riled up: the new thinking that the "pelvic exam" (the speculum and exam by hand) isn't necessary unless a woman reports problematic symptoms. In fact, the most recent recommendations from the U.S. Preventive Services Task Force (USPSTF) state: "No good- or fair-quality studies directly evaluated the effectiveness of screening pelvic examinations in asymptomatic—no noticeable problems—non-pregnant adult women to improve quality of life, reduce disease-specific morbidity, or reduce disease-specific or all-cause mortality." In laymen speak, there's no definitive proof that an annual pelvic exam is necessary to have a long, healthy life with your lady parts.

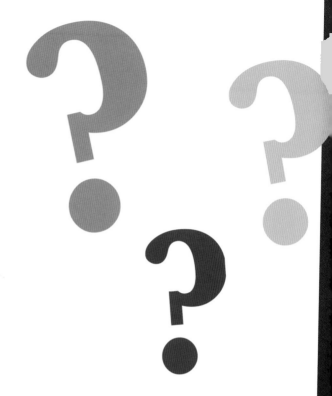

Okay, that's them—and their findings deserve mentioning. But the American College of Obstetricians and Gynecologists (ACOG) recommends "performing pelvic examinations annually in all patients age 21 years and older." While the ACOG, like the USPSTF, found no evidence to support or refute the benefit of an annual pelvic examination (meaning speculum and bimanual examination) in asymptomatic, low-risk (read: overall healthy) patients, it did conclude that the decision to perform a complete examination at the annual wellness visit should be a shared decision between the patient and the gyno.

So what's a gyno to do? What are you to do? My recommendation is that a preventive visit is valuable. Whether an actual pelvic exam is needed or not should be decided on an individual basis.

And what about the Pap portion of the exam? Should that be done annually? In fact, for many healthy ladies, a Pap test is only needed every three years from age 21 to 29, followed by every three for women aged 30 to 65, including an HPV test every five years at the very least.

But it should also be emphasized that a gyno visit is soooooo much more than just a pelvic exam and Pap test. Even if you're in a year that doesn't require these tests, an annual well-woman visit allows your doc to address so many other things—especially if you're one of the many women for whom the gyno is the only doc you see (I don't recommend this, but it's often the case).

Your OB/GYN should always (no exceptions) be sensitive and nonjudgmental—no topic is off limits. Really!

—Dr. Dweck

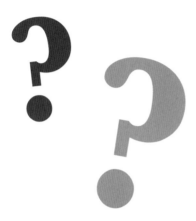

WHY WE GO TO THE GYNO (BESIDES OUR ANNUAL EXAM)

- Vaginal discharge
- Abnormal bleeding
- Pain
- Urinary complaints
- Breast problems
- Sex issues
- Problems getting pregnant

Note: According to the ACOG, lesbians may be at higher risk for certain cancers (colon, lung, uterine, ovarian, and breast), cardiovascular disease, and diabetes but, in general, should be screened according to standard guidelines. Also, STDs can be transmitted between women.

HOW YOUNG IS OLD ENOUGH FOR THE FIRST TRIP TO THE GYNO?

According to the recommendation of the American College of Obstetricians and Gynecologists (ACOG), little women should have their first exam when they are between 13 and 15 years old (sooner if they're sexually active). The initial visit won't necessarily include a pelvic examination, but the doctor will provide guidance, preventive services, and screening. The ACOG recommends annual screening for gonorrhea for all sexually active adolescents and for chlamydia in all sexually active women 25 and younger. (See the prior page for Pap test guidelines.) Hopefully, there will be a connection with the doctor, so contacting him or her will feel comfortable, easy, and necessary should any problems pop up in the future.

A NOTE ON CONFIDENTIALITY Adolescents may undergo a pelvic examination without their parents' knowledge or permission if the exam is performed for the testing or treatment of a sexually transmitted disease. Laws vary by jurisdiction regarding confidential access to HIV testing, contraception, and abortion services. Parental consent is required for childhood examinations and adolescent pelvic exams unrelated to sexual contact.

H

IS FOR HORMONES DURING MENOPAUSE

How to Tell When You're in It—
Hot Flashes, Jalapeno Peppers, and More

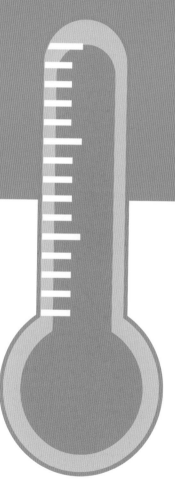

Menopause is a touchy subject for lots of us careening toward what can be bumpy terrain or already jostling through it. Of course some lucky sisters are clueless and breeze along, but let's not talk about them right now. There are more than 19 million American women driving through menopause this year, and it's predicted that by 2025, 1.1 billion women in the world will be going through it. Wow! And for plenty of those ladies, it will feel like maneuvering a Mack truck. Hold on to that wheel!

HOT FLASHES SHOULD REALLY BE CALLED AWESOME POWER SURGES!!!

If scientists ever find a cure for menopause, our big problem will be global cooling.

SO, WHAT IS MENOPAUSE?

Okay, let me explain without any hype: It's a time in your life, usually between the ages of 45 and 55, when your ovaries stop producing estrogen and your menstrual period ends. The average age of menopause is 51. Sound simple? Well . . . there are also other terms that are sometimes used to describe the time before and after you stop menstruating:

PERIMENOPAUSE The menopause transition starts when your menstrual periods first begin to change. They can become more or less frequent with more or less bleeding, including skipped periods, and this transition can last for upwards of ten years. Perimenopause can begin in a woman's early forties.

MENOPAUSE Clinically, it is diagnosed as 12 straight months of amenorrhea (no period) in a woman over 40 if there aren't any other causes. It is a diagnosis often made in hindsight.

POSTMENOPAUSE The time after menopause.

IS THERE ANY WAY TO KNOW WHEN I'M GOING TO GO THROUGH MENOPAUSE?

Got a crystal ball? Actually you won't need one. Though defining the actual moment you enter menopause is impossible, there are factors that can affect its timing and onset:

GENETIC If the women in your family have gone through an early menopause, you're also likely to go through it sooner.

LIFESTYLE The age of menopause is reduced by about two years in women who smoke.

FACTOID Sixty-five percent of the women surveyed at the Social Issues Research Centre in England, aged 50 to 64, reported being happier after menopause than before; 66 percent were more independent, and 59 percent were enjoying better relationships with their partners and friends.

I THINK I'M IN IT; WHAT SHOULD I DO NEXT?

Don't murder your partner. Only kidding . . . sort of.

Seriously, if you're over 40 and haven't had a menstrual period in 12 months, there's a good chance you're in menopause. Most women don't need lab testing to confirm it, especially if they are having symptoms such as hot flashes, night sweats, or vaginal dryness. Hormonal lab tests such as FSH or estradiol may be helpful in diagnosis, but they won't necessarily give a surefire answer because hormones that are being tested have levels that vary month-to-month during perimenopause.

I'VE HAD A HYSTERECTOMY. WILL I GO THROUGH MENOPAUSE?

After a hysterectomy (see more about this on page 88), when you no longer have a uterus (but still have ovaries), it can be tougher to know if you're menopausal because you're not menstruating. You might develop menopausal symptoms as your ovaries stop working and the levels of estrogen in your blood begin to fall. If you have bothersome symptoms of menopause after a hysterectomy, give your doctor a buzz. This scenario also applies to women who have stopped menstruating because they've had a uterine ablation (a procedure done by your gynecologist to treat heavy bleeding in which the uterus is left in place, but the lining that proliferates and bleeds each month is obliterated; the ovaries are left untouched and they're not affected by the procedure).

FAST FACT There are only three female animals known to go through menopause: elephants, humpback whales, and humans.

MY PERIOD IS SO WACKY! I JUST WANT TO KNOW IF I'M OKAY.

The majority of ladies begin to notice changes in their periods during perimenopause. If this means you, relax, changes are normal and might include:

- having your period more or less often than usual (a typical cycle length is 21 to 45 days)

- bleeding for fewer days than before

- skipping one or more periods

FROM THE FILE OF STUPID JOKES
Q: How do you assume the mood of your menopausal wife?
A: Assume her mood is lousy, and occasionally you'll be wrong.

NOT-SO-FAST FACT

Are you a red-hot mama? The conventional wisdom is that the majority of women who experience hot flashes are over the heat hump within 18 to 24 months. But hold on! For some unlucky ladies, hot flashes can continue for many years, and the earlier they begin, the longer a woman is likely to suffer, according to the Study of Women's Health Across the Nation (SWAN) published in *JAMA Internal Medicine*. In a racially, ethnically, and geographically diverse group of women with frequent hot flashes or night sweats (the largest study to date), the median length of time women endured symptoms was 7.4 years. So, while half of the women were affected for less than that time, half had symptoms longer—some for 14 years, according to the study.

HOW CAN I TELL IF I'M BLEEDING TOO MUCH?

Sometimes it's hard to know whether you're on over-flow, but for perimenopausal women, it's an important thing to keep an eye on this as the risk of cancer goes up with age. It's a good idea to see your doctor if you're bleeding

- more often than every three weeks

- excessively and it's interfering with your life

- between periods—even if only spotting

- after menopause (even if it's just a dot)

- after sex

NOTE: Irregular vaginal bleeding may be a normal part of menopause, or it may be a sign of pregnancy, thyroid disease, or something else—another reason to check in with your gyno.

I'M IN PERIMENOPAUSE. DO I STILL NEED BIRTH CONTROL?

Don't dump your birth control pills or pull your IUD yet. Sure, you're less likely to get pregnant after 45, but it's possible—especially if you're still having occasional periods and having sex regularly. And, dudette, if you don't want to be pregnant, you should continue to use some form of birth control until you're positively menopausal. Wishful thinking doesn't count.

HOT FLASHES

These sizzling bolts of fire typically begin as a sudden sensation of heat centered in your upper chest and face and spread fast through your body. This burning sensation can last from two to four minutes, is often associated with profuse perspiration and occasionally palpitations, and is sometimes followed by chills and shivering and/or a feeling of anxiety. And don't think they're just a flash in the pan. Hot flashes usually occur several times a day; some women get only one or two each day while others suffer dozens of them; some women get them nonstop day and night. When flashes happen at night, they frequently interfere with sleep. But hey, some women don't get any!

Additional factors related to longer duration of hot flashes and night sweats are younger age at onset, greater perceived stress, greater sensitivity to these symptoms, and higher depressive symptoms.

THINGS THAT STOKE THE FLAMES OF HOT FLASHES

- Smoking

- High body mass index: Overweight women are more likely to have hot flashes.

- Little to no physical activity

- Stress

- Caffeine

- Poor diet

- Alcohol consumption, particularly red wine

- Consuming MSG

- Eating big meals

FYI If you're in your forties and you stop having periods, or if you have questions about menopausal symptoms, speak to your doctor. You may need further testing to see if another issue, including pregnancy, is the reason for your symptoms.

FACTOID In the Western world, about 75 to 85 percent of women experience hot flashes. African American women reported the longest duration (median of 10.1 years) and Japanese and Chinese women had the shortest duration (median of 4.8 years and 5.4 years, respectively). The median total durations were 6.5 years for non-Hispanic white women and 8.9 years for Hispanic women.

IT FEELS LIKE I HAVE A FEVER AT NIGHT, AND MY SHEETS GET SOAKED. WHAT'S GOING ON?

When hot flashes happen during sleep, they're called night sweats. These steamy "darlings" may make you perspire through your clothes and wake up because you're either hot or cold (because the sweat is evaporating). This can happen one or more times a night. And truthfully, Ms. Groggy, a good night's sleep, which you aren't getting, is crucial for your mental and physical well-being. Thank your crummy night's sleep if you develop other problems such as fatigue, irritability, trouble concentrating, and mood swings. It can be a nightmare.

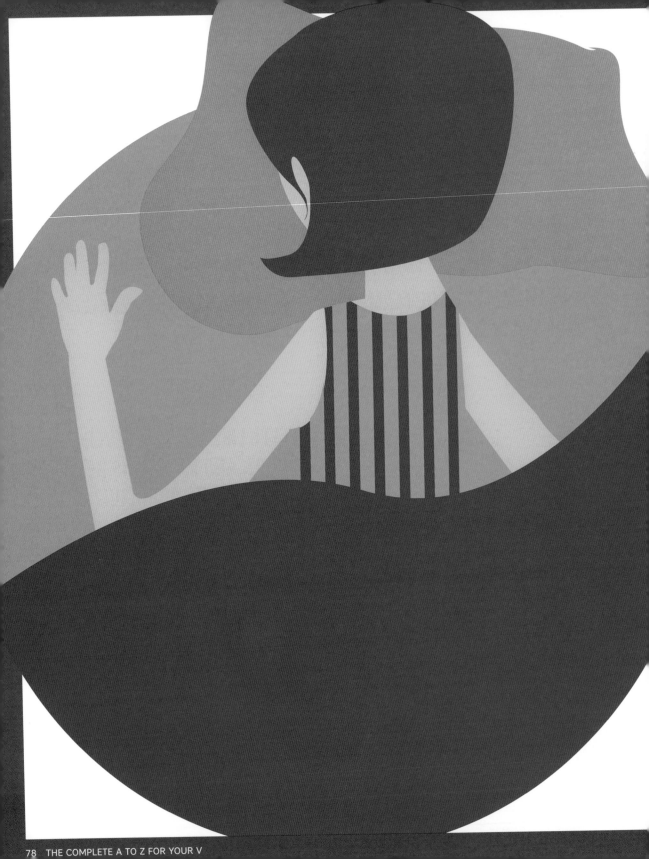

EASY, SUPER COOL WAYS TO STOP HOT FLASHES

- Dress in layers that you can shed when flashes arise. Don't wear wool or synthetics, and be wary of silk. Avoid turtlenecks; stick to open-neck shirts.

- Keep ice water at hand and nix hot beverages. Substitute caffeine-free soft drinks or seltzer for alcohol.

- Reduce or eliminate caffeine.

- Pass on jalapenos! Also avoid cayenne, chili peppers, wasabi, and hot mustard. Spicy foods can easily bring on hot flashes.

- Eat smaller, more frequent meals rather than large ones.

- Lower the thermostat.

- Wear pajamas or a nightgown that is cotton and loose fitting to wick away moisture, or just your birthday suit, to bed.

- Use cotton, not synthetic, sheets.

- Get a bigger bed if you and your partner are on different heat planets.

- Take a cool shower before bed.

- Leave the bed and stick your head in the freezer. Trust me!

OMG. I'M SO DRY DOWN THERE!

Well, sadly that's one of the side effects of menopause. As levels of estrogen in your blood fall, tissues inside your vagina and urethra can become thin, delicate, inelastic, and dry. But you can:

GET JUICY WITHOUT HORMONES

Caveat: Most suggestions require a few weeks to work, so be patient!

- Boost your water intake.

- Avoid heavy fragrances and harsh chemicals in personal hygiene products.

- Eat soy and other foods containing "plant estrogens."

- Try an over-the-counter personal moisturizer such as Replens or Lubrigyn.

CELEBRATE! October 18 is World Menopause Day.

FROM THE OH-NO-WHAT-ELSE? FILES

- **BALANCE** You can probably blame an estrogen deficiency if you're off-kilter during menopause.
- **SKIN CHANGES** Collagen in the skin and bones is reduced by estrogen deficiency and can lead to aging and wrinkling of the skin.
- **JOINT PAIN** Some women experience diffuse joint pain during menopausal transition and the postmenopausal period.
- **MENSTRUAL MIGRAINES** These headaches cluster around the onset of each menstrual period. Women hope they'll stop once they are menopausal, but no such luck. In many women, these headaches may worsen in frequency and intensity during the transition (perimenopause).
- **BREAST PAIN** Tenderness and pain are common during early menopause but begin to lessen in the later transition.

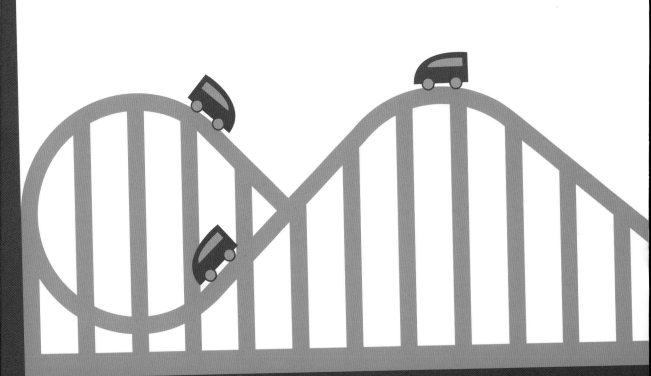

I ONCE LOVED TO HAVE SEX, NOW I COULDN'T CARE LESS. WHAT'S WRONG WITH ME?

Probably nothing. Vaginal dryness can lead to pain with sex. And just the fear of this pain can result in a lower sex drive. Good news! Some women report regaining their sex drive once they are postmenopausal, even without replacement hormones. Why? No fear of pregnancy and no issues with that time of the month!

Dare we mention the laundry list of what might also be going on here?

- Hormonal fluctuations including lower testosterone thus lower libido

- Relationship issues

- Sexual boredom

- Fatigue and exhaustion

- Confounding medical issues and/or medications

- General life stress and the blahs

- Poor body image and sexual self-esteem, especially if you're not feeling like a beauty queen. And who does?

But guess what? Perimenopausal women often enjoy a "surge" in libido because of hormonal fluctuations.

WHY AM I ON AN EMOTIONAL ROLLER COASTER?

Some menopausal and perimenopausal ladies develop problems with mood, such as sadness, difficulty concentrating, feeling uninterested in normal activities, and sleeping too much or having trouble staying asleep. Try getting plenty of natural sunlight (don't forget the sunscreen!), avoid alcohol, exercise, and try talk therapy with friends or a professional. Also, let your doctor know if you're experiencing more than the blahs.

HOW ABOUT HORMONE REPLACEMENT THERAPY (HRT)?

HRT includes estrogen and progestin to ease some symptoms of menopause, ranging from hot flashes to preventing osteoporosis. While HRT or ERT (when only estrogen is used) can drastically improve the quality of life for some women, others don't suffer symptoms to warrant treatment.

Despite all the good that hormone therapy can do, you've probably also heard there is a lot of controversy around it. As with all medications, there are health risks, and as the number of risks associated with hormone therapy are increasingly recognized, docs are less likely to prescribe it and plenty of sisters are discontinuing its use. That said, get the facts first and then discuss your individual situation with your gyno. The pendulum has swung slightly again: HRT/ERT is now being considered for women whose quality of life is severely lessened by menopausal symptoms. Now the common rule of thumb is that HRT is a reasonable treatment at its lowest dose for the shortest amount of time possible based on symptom severity and other individual circumstances.

CAUTION You should NOT take hormone replacement if you have a history of blood clots, breast cancer, or heart disease. Also, you probably don't need to take hormones if menopausal symptoms aren't bothering you.

SO, WHAT ARE THE BENEFITS OF HRT?

The most common reason to take hormone therapy is to treat those loathsome menopausal symptoms we've been talking about. Women who opt for standard hormone therapy during menopause are typically prescribed estrogen and progestin. Beyond alleviating symptoms, benefits include protection from osteoporosis, colorectal cancer, and symptoms of vaginal atrophy (also known as the genitourinary symptoms of menopause, or GSM, meaning the signs and symptoms that occur in the vagina during menopause, including vaginal dryness, burning, itching, pallor, delicate tissue, loss of elasticity, urinary frequency or discomfort, painful intercourse, and more).

IS THERE ANY WAY TO REDUCE HRT'S RISKS?

- Minimize the amount of medication you take. Use the lowest effective dose for the shortest amount of time needed to treat symptoms.

- Find the best delivery method for you. You can take estrogen in the form of a pill, patch, gel, vaginal cream, pill, or ring.

- Use progestin. If you haven't had a hysterectomy and are using systemic estrogen therapy, you will also need progestin to protect you from developing uterine cancer.

ARE THERE ANY MEDICATIONS BESIDES HRT THAT HELP RELIEVE MENOPAUSAL SYMPTOMS?

- SSRIs, antidepressants such as Prozac, Zoloft, and Effexor.

- Antianxiety meds such as Xanax can reduce anxiety and help with sleep. Note: These meds are habit forming. Use with caution.

- Clonidine is an antihypertensive pill or patch that can relieve hot flashes.

- Progesterone may help reduce hot flashes. Added bonus: Prometrium (micronized bioidentical) progesterone makes you sleepy—take it before bed and it's a win-win: fewer hot flashes and better sleep. Caution: Avoid this med if you are allergic to peanuts.

I've got postmenopausal zest!

—Margaret Mead

MY FRIEND IS USING SOMETHING CALLED BIOIDENTICAL HORMONE THERAPY. DOES IT REALLY WORK?

Bioidentical hormones have a chemical structure similar to the hormones that the human body naturally produces. They claim to create similar results to HRT and ERT, and are sometimes touted as more "natural." The treatment involves individual doses of compounded (made specifically for you at a specialized pharmacy) or pharmaceutical-company-produced medications that come in patches, pills, gels, sublingual tablets, even suppositories. Speak with your doctor about what this therapy involves. Bummer alert: There's no evidence that bioidentical hormone therapy is any safer or more effective than traditional HRT.

FAST FACT According to the North American Menopause Society, more than 30 percent of women say they use herbal remedies and supplements such as evening primrose oil, black cohosh, and red clover to deal with their symptoms.

WHAT ABOUT PHYTOESTROGENS?

Big word but not a big help. Plant-derived estrogens are called phytoestrogens. They have been marketed as a "safer" alternative to hormones for women with menopausal symptoms. The effectiveness of supplements containing phytoestrogens such as red clover, black cohash, or evening primrose oil is questionable, although some women claim anecdotally that they help. Women who have had breast cancer should avoid supplemental phytoestrogens. Because phytoestrogens are found in so many healthful foods such as soybeans, tofu and other dietary soy, chickpeas, lentils, flaxseed, grains, fruits and vegetables, I recommend making these foods part of your diet instead of taking processed supplements.

I

IS FOR INTERCOURSE ISSUES

All the Snafus That Can Happen to You and What You Can Do About Them

According to surveys, the Americans and Greeks top the list of intercourse frequency, doing it on average 124 and 117 times each year, respectively. The Indians do it only about 76 times a year, while the Japanese seem to be the least interested, clocking in at a lowly 36 times annually.

There are approximately 100 million acts of sexual intercourse around the world each day.

AND HOW MANY OF THOSE ACTS ARE AWESOME?

While sex can be one of the most loving and fun activities you can engage in, that doesn't mean it always goes well. When it's great, it's great, and there are countless ways it can be great. On the other hand, there are a number of issues that can prevent you from having all the O's you want. The good news is that many of these snafus are totally treatable. Rather than beat around the bush, if having sexual intercourse is no longer fun, or was never a bowl of cherries, read on to see what might be going on—and perhaps discover you're far from alone.

VAGINAL DRYNESS

It can happen at any age, although it's most common in postmenopausal women. Some reasons why we go dry are:
- declining estrogen levels
- inhibited desire
- inadequate foreplay
- medications such as antihistamines, antidepressants, and antihypertensives
- medical disorders such as diabetes, thyroid disorders, and heart disease

NOW FOR THE GOOD NEWS: DRYNESS CAN BE MANAGED!
Here are some tips on how to get wet:
- Increase foreplay to give more time for natural lubrication.
- Hold off penetration until you're driven mad by yearning.
- Try OTC vaginal moisturizers and lubricants. Daily vaginal moisturizers like Replens don't contain hormones. OTC lubricants to use during sex include K-Y Jelly, Astroglide, and Überlube. Follow directions.
- Give natural lubricants like coconut oil a whirl.
- Avoid perfumed body or hand lotions, which may be irritating to the vagina.
- Speak with your gyno about vaginal estrogen, which requires a prescription and may not be right for every woman, but can work very well for the right candidates. Vaginal estrogen comes in various forms: creams, rings, and tablets. Vagifem, for instance, is a small vaginal estrogen tablet inserted twice weekly. There is also Estring, a flexible vaginal ring worn inside the vagina for three months at a time. Both products claim minimal to no absorption of estrogen into the bloodstream—and therefore carry little risk of breast cancer and blood clots. In fact, minimally absorbed vaginal estrogen has recently been given the go-ahead as a reasonable solution to painful sex due to dryness even for women with a history of breast cancer if non-hormonal options fail. That said, each circumstance is different and very personal.

Remember, use it or lose it! Sexual activity, including masturbation, may help the vaginal tissues remain elastic and soft and prevent narrowing and discomfort.

> *No woman needs intercourse; few women escape it.*
>
> —Andrea Dworkin, Feminist

SEMEN ALLERGY

Sometimes sisters complain about itching, burning, swelling, and redness, and, much less commonly, shortness of breath, rash, and hives that last an hour or so after sexual intercourse. On exam there's no sign of infection, skin condition, or reaction to a particular product. In these unusual cases, patients have asked, "Could I be allergic to my partner?" The short answer is yes—and most often women under 40 years old with a family history of major allergic reactions are complaining. Talk about an intimacy obstacle! Since symptoms won't occur if condoms are used, that's one way to prevent them. Another, in severe cases, is medication. You could pre-dose with antihistamines. The downside? You might fall asleep in the middle of making love. So, speak with your doc.

VAGINISMUS

Otherwise known as genito-pelvic pain/penetration disorder (GPPPD), this is a tightening and spasming of the muscles at your V's opening. This involuntary muscle contraction can make it painful, difficult, or virtually impossible to have vaginal intercourse. In fact, vaginismus can also make putting in a tampon or a pelvic exam tough going. You can get your lady flower to blossom using a vaginal dilator that gradually increases the size, through physical therapy and relaxation exercises, and even by intravaginal Valium.

VULVODYNIA

This is an unprovoked stinging, burning, irritation, rawness, or pain anywhere on the vulva that occurs during intercourse, from tactile stimulation, or even spontaneously with no obvious cause. Your gyno will diagnose your condition based on your history and a physical exam and by cancelling out all the other usual suspects. Treatment is an individual matter. It may include application of topical anesthetic jelly ten minutes before sexual intercourse (don't forget to wipe away the excess prior to sex so that your partner's penis doesn't go numb!), meticulous hygiene, hypoallergenic lubricants, physical therapy, Botox injections, antidepressants, analgesics (pain meds), nerve blocks, and of course emotional support and counseling. Vulvar ice packs are also soothing after sex. You can find more helpful information through the National Vulvodynia Association at www.nva.org.

FROM THE NO-MATTER-HOW-YOU-SAY-IT FILES: screw, bang, reproduce, copulate, pork, boogie, hump your honey, get laid, lay some pipe, hide the salami, bury the bone, stuff the donut, dine in the Y, munch on the rug, or whack Willy Wonka into Wonderland . . .

DEEP PAIN

Sometimes pain felt deep inside during sex might be due to your individual anatomy and can be managed by simply changing positions. For example, if your uterus is tilted, missionary position may be uncomfortable but being on top could feel much better. However, this type of pain could signal other issues, so discussing it with your gyno is essential. It could be one of these conditions:

PELVIC INFLAMMATORY DISEASE (PID) is an infection of the uterus, fallopian tubes, and nearby pelvic structures that can cause scar tissue and chronic pelvic pain including pain during sex. Treatment involves antibiotics and at times surgery.

OVARIAN CYSTS are diagnosed through medical history, a physical exam, and an ultrasound. Treatment may include expectant management (watching and waiting), medication, birth control pills (which can suppress ovarian cysts), or surgery for definitive removal.

FIBROIDS are benign muscular growths on the uterus and are common. They are a frequent cause of discomfort during sex. For some women, fibroids are small and no problem. Other women hold off on treatment because fibroids usually shrink in menopause. In some

SISTERS WITH V ABNORMALITIES FROM BIRTH or because of trauma or women who have undergone female circumcision may benefit from surgical treatment to enhance the vagina for better sexual function. Sexual abuse is associated with chronic pelvic pain and sexual pain disorders. If this is true for you, seek counseling and therapy. There's an excellent chance you can be helped.

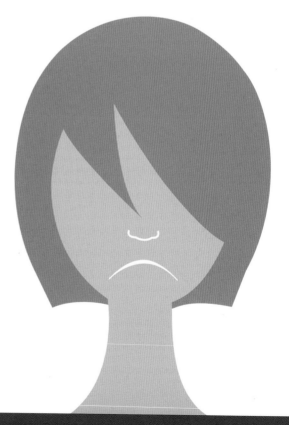

cases, however, fibroids cause unmanageable symptoms including heavy bleeding. In these cases, options include surgical removal with myomectomy (removal of fibroids only), hysterectomy (removal of the uterus with fibroids), or embolization, an invasive procedure to diminish the blood supply to the uterus in an effort to shrink fibroids.

ENDOMETRIOSIS A condition in which cells that typically line the uterus are found on your ovaries, fallopian tubes, and other pelvic structures. This tissue then bleeds monthly due to hormonal changes and can cause scarring and pain. Diagnosis is made by history (the condition tends to run in families), physical exam, and at times laparoscopy.

GENITAL PROLAPSE When the cervix, uterus, vagina, bladder, or rectum is bulging inside or protruding from the vagina. It can be brought on by childbirth, being overweight, or genetic predisposition. While Kegel exercises may help in very mild cases, surgical intervention

DIET DELIGHT Sex can burn about 70 to 120 calories for a 130-pound woman and 77 to 155 calories for a 170-pound man every hour.

may be necessary in severe cases. A common treatment option for prolapse includes insertion of a pessary, which is a firm rubber device with support, to hold the organs inside. Unfortunately, such a device means sexual intercourse is O-U-T. Fortunately, a new, totally cool alternative called the Elvie is now available. This vaginal device, a sort of Fitbit for the pelvic floor, acts as a personal trainer for your pelvic-floor muscles. It even comes with Bluetooth capabilities and a phone app that provides biofeedback so that you can check on your progress.

HYSTERECTOMY AND SEXUAL INTERCOURSE

A hysterectomy, which is the surgical removal of the uterus, does not generally affect sexual function after you've healed. But here's a caveat: If your ovaries are removed as well, your estrogen will be depleted and then dryness will occur. Some surgeons and patients feel that retaining the cervix during hysterectomy may make for better sexual function and pelvic support.

Here's the conundrum: The reason for hysterectomy may impact one's sex life more than the surgery itself. It's personal. Women undergoing surgery for cancer may be depressed, fatigued, and facing further treatment. Others are so happy and relieved to have treated heavy bleeding or large fibroids, for example, with a hysterectomy that they feel liberated and actually have a better sex life after the operation.

J

IS FOR JUST NOT TRUE

Junking the Misinformation,
Misconceptions, and Myths
That Confuse Us All

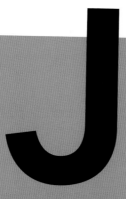

Yada yada yada. Sisters love to talk. We share our deepest secrets and we're quick to offer advice and know-how about what we know about—and what we don't really know about. That's a big part of what brings us together, keeps us solid, and makes us cool. But stuff goes wrong: Sometimes a personal anecdote becomes dyed-in-the-wool truth when, in fact, it's only one woman's personal story. Or we convey something as absolutely, definitely true, when there is only a little "truthiness" to it, meaning there's a trace of fact but it's pretty muddy. Or we repeat the same old wives' tales we heard from our mothers. Not that we're dissing our mothers. It's more like the old game of telephone: Info gets distorted the more it's repeated.

Disinformation is duping. Misinformation is tricking.

—Toba Beta, *Master of Stupidity*

The mission of this chapter is to take care of all this misinformation, right here, right now. Let's dig into the most common misconceptions that come up over and over again in Dr. Dweck's day-to-day practice.

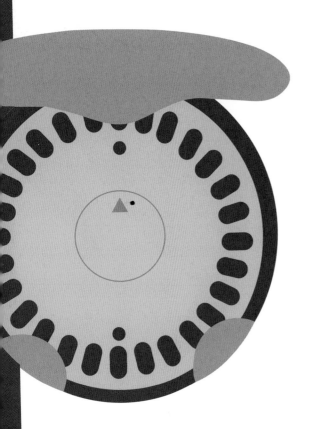

LIES ABOUT BIRTH CONTROL PILLS

LIE: YOU NEED TO TAKE A BREAK FROM THE BIRTH CONTROL PILL AT LEAST ONCE A YEAR.

Heck no. Many women can safely stay on the pill until menopause without a break.

LIE: USING THE PILL MAY MAKE IT HARDER TO GET PREGNANT IN THE FUTURE.

Relax. The pill won't harm your fertility or prevent you from getting pregnant in the future. A couple of caveats: If you went on the pill to control irregular cycles, you might still have irregular cycles when you get off the pill. For this reason, you might have trouble conceiving because you may have a preexisting ovulation issue. Also, if you're over 35 when you stop taking the pill, your fertility is likely to have declined due to age. Eggs only last so long!

LIE: YOU NEED TO WAIT THREE MONTHS AFTER COMING OFF THE PILL TO CONCEIVE.

Nah. You don't have to wait any specific amount of time after stopping the pill in order to conceive safely. The only reason it may be recommended to wait three months is that it could take that long for your cycle to regulate, and it may be easier to date your pregnancy. But the truth is, there is no harm in trying right away.

LIE: IT'S UNSAFE TO USE THE PILL TO MANIPULATE YOUR CYCLE.

It's perfectly safe and docs have been recommending this method for years. For example, if you don't want to get your period on your wedding day, honeymoon, or vacation, or at an athletic event, you can skip the placebo days of the pill and start a new pack as soon as you finish the last hormone pill in your current pack. This will keep you from getting your period that month, but keep in mind you can occasionally get breakthrough bleeding when manipulating your pills. You can do similar manipulations with other hormone birth controls such as the patch or ring. Ask your gyno for instructions if you feel at all unclear on how to make an effective skip happen.

LIE: THE PILL ALWAYS CAUSES HUGE WEIGHT GAIN.

Here's an example of truthiness: Some ladies do gain weight on the pill, but most ladies don't. If you are one of the gainers, it's probably only due to water retention, and you will likely gain no more than two to three pounds (about 1 kilogram) of water weight. The myth of weight gain may come from the fact that many girls start the pill during adolescence or when going off to college, which are times when healthy young women gain some weight anyway. So, in this instance, packing on the pounds is just a timely coincidence. Some women, however, do find that the pill bumps up their appetite, and if they don't pump up their willpower, they could be digging into a nightly bag of chips. If this is your scenario, ask your gyno to try switching you to a different brand of birth control pill.

LIES ABOUT SEX, AND CONCEPTION, AND STDS

LIE: YOU CAN'T GET PREGNANT IF A MAN PULLS OUT PRIOR TO EJACULATION.

Don't take any chances. It's possible there's sperm in the pre-ejaculate fluid your guy secretes before he climaxes.

LIE: USING LUBRICANT WILL HELP YOU TO GET PREGNANT.

This is totally false. Some lubricants can actually prevent you from getting pregnant. If you're really dry and trying to conceive, be creative. Opt for a sperm-friendly OTC lubricant such as Pre-Seed.

LIE: CONDOMS PREVENT THE TRANSMISSION OF ALL STDS.

While it's less likely you'll get an STD when condoms are used, you're still vulnerable to transmission. HPV and herpes in particular can be spread by direct contact with areas not covered by the condom.

BUT DON'T BE A FOOL, VULCANIZE THE TOOL!

LIE: ONLY WOMEN WHO HAVE HAD CASUAL SEX CAN GET STDS.

Seriously, you only have to have unprotected sex one time just once with one partner who has had other partners to potentially be exposed to STDs. And remember: Some STDs can be spread via oral and anal sex as well as skin-to-skin contact.

FOUR MORE NO-WAY-JOSE MYTHS

1. The HPV vaccine (Gardasil) causes HPV. Just the opposite: This vaccine protects against nine strains of HPV that are causes of cervical, oropharyngeal, and anal cancers.
2. Condoms are reusable. In fact, you should never be stingy with the condom. You also need to grab a new one if you're switching between vaginal and anal sex. And vice versa.
3. The pill is only for young peeps. Many perimenopausal women are great candidates for the pill barring some medical issues or smoking habits (smoking increases the pill's risks). Speak with the doc.
4. You can't get herpes from oral sex. Oral-genital transmission is definitely possible.

LIE: IN A MONOGAMOUS RELATIONSHIP, AN HPV DIAGNOSIS ALWAYS MEANS SOMEONE HAS CHEATED.

Stop the divorce papers! An HPV diagnosis may be the result of a persistent but previously undiagnosed HPV infection from years (even decades) ago rather than a new exposure.

LIE: INTERCOURSE DURING PREGNANCY IS DANGEROUS FOR THE BABY.

Intercourse is safe during pregnancy—unless your doc has nixed it. Your babe is well protected inside your muscular uterus and is cushioned in cozy fluid.

LIE: THE MORNING-AFTER PILL CAUSES ABORTIONS.

In fact, emergency contraception prevents pregnancy by blocking fertilization and implantation. It does not induce abortions.

LIE: IF YOU'RE A VIRGIN, YOU HAVE A HYMEN.

Sure, some women "break" their hymen when they first have intercourse—but lots of other sisters break theirs by bike riding or horseback riding or by some other vigorous activity. And these women don't always bleed profusely, either.

LIE: SIMULTANEOUS ORGASMS ARE A MUST FOR A GREAT SEX LIFE.

No way. Women can see stars, hear whistles blowing, and fly to the metaphorical moon while having orgasm after orgasm while their partner just relishes in giving them. Or they can enjoy sex to the max without even having an orgasm. One thing is for sure: It really doesn't depend on synchronicity.

Q: Are birth control pills tax deductible?
A: Only if they don't work.

The priceless galaxy of misinformation called the mind.

—Djuna Barnes

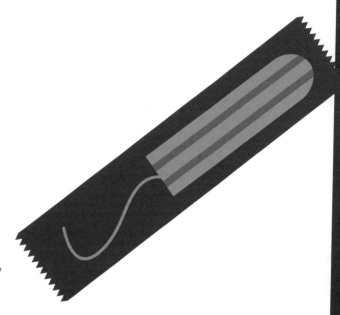

LIES ABOUT YOUR PERIOD

LIE: YOU SHOULDN'T EXERCISE OR DO STRENUOUS ACTIVITY DURING YOUR PERIOD.

Just do it. There's no harm in exercising while you've got your period. Bonus points: It may even help with cramps.

LIE: EVERYONE CAN SEE YOUR PAD!

This is a lie we tell ourselves, because we can be super aware of wearing a pad sometimes. Rest assured, though, that even if it feels bulky to you, it is incredibly unlikely that anyone can see it.

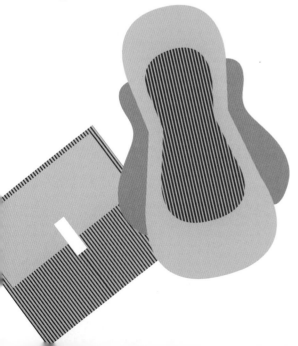

LIE: IF YOU HAVE AN IUD, YOU CAN'T USE TAMPONS.

Some women worry that if they pull out a tampon, the IUD will also come out. But that's not true. An IUD does not interfere with tampons.

LIE: YOU CAN'T HAVE YOUR PERIOD AND A YEAST INFECTION OR BV (BACTERIAL VAGINOSIS) AT THE SAME TIME.

All these things can overlap, and in fact sometimes the hormonal changes that happen right before a period can bring on a yeast infection in some women. The good news: These infections can clear up on their own after a period due to changes in vaginal pH.

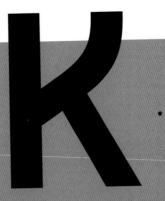

K

IS FOR KILLER EXERCISES

Infection-Inducing Activities, Problematic
Pastimes, and How to Recover from All
Sorts of Cha-Cha Trauma

Exercise isn't supposed to be bad for you,
right? Right! You put all this time, energy, and
effort into exercising because it's supposed to
be really good for your body, self-esteem, and
mental state. Then lo and behold, it's crushing
your lovely lady bits or causing infections or
even sores. Well, it doesn't have to be this way!
For each exercise endeavor, there's a way to
make it better for your delicate lady flower.

ALL THIS RUNNING IS RUINING MY VAJAYJAY!

We are talking about some major chafing here. This is a real problem for runners, especially in warm weather or with longer distances. Sweaty clothing and skin rubbing against skin can cause painful stinging or burning and a red rash. It's most common around the groin and inner thighs—and the nipples. (Okay, so nipples aren't related to the V but this is really awful and common, so it's worth mentioning.) Tighter-fitting and moisture-wicking or cotton clothing will help to prevent chafing. Before running, try applying A+D ointment, Vaseline, cornstarch, or Udder Balm (yes, it's typically used for cow udders; we're not saying you're a cow but, hey, it works). Smearing one of these products externally on the vulva, groin, and inner thighs (never inside the vagina) may prevent chafing.

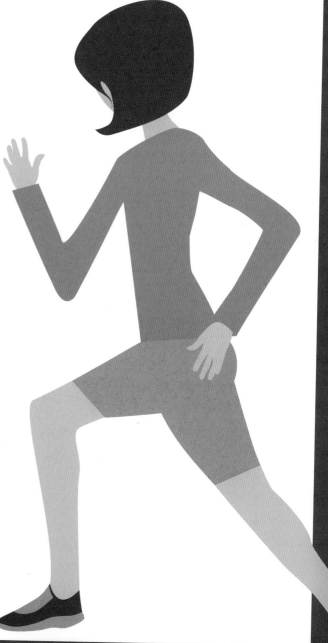

GENERAL RULE Hydrate well and get out of damp and wet workout clothes and swimsuits as soon as possible to avoid vulvar infection, irritation, and V infection.

FROM THE STRANGE-BUT-TRUE MEDICAL FILES
Changing a lightbulb can cause damage to your lady flower! While a patient was standing on a chair to change a lightbulb she fell, hitting her V on the back post of the chair!

I'VE BEEN TRAINING FOR A CENTURY BIKE RIDE AND IT'S REALLY BOTHERING MY V AREA. I SWEAR I'M NOT ONLY FEELING SORE, I'M GETTING SORES!

Ooh, the irritation, discomfort, and at times pressure sores (with cracked and broken skin or blisters) that can happen to your poor vulva thanks to cycling. Not surprisingly, these are commonly known as "saddle sores." Girl, they can be a pain in the ass—I mean, pain in the vajayjay. Prevention is in order: Padded chamois shorts are a must whenever you're cycling or spinning. Consider a gel seat cover for more padding and cushioning. An open seat with V cut out or groove or an ultra-wide cushiony cruiser seat may help to prevent pressure sores. A biking balm, such as Chamois Butt'r or Bodyglide, can be applied to high-friction areas or shorts to limit chafing and reduce saddle sores—especially helpful if you're going on a long ride.

I THINK SWIMMING IS GIVING ME A YEAST INFECTION.

I'll bet you're staying in your wet swimsuit for an extended period of time, perhaps lolling poolside with a piña colada in hand? Well, while you're enjoying yourself, a vulvar and vaginal infection or irritation can be developing. Get out of that suit and into something dry and sexy before you schmooze! Oh, and while we're on the subject of swimming, don't worry about swimming while you're menstruating. Swimming with a tampon in shouldn't cause a problem. And forget old wives' tales: It's unlikely menstrual blood will attract sharks while scuba diving or snorkeling. Your blood is still in your body, just like with every body at all points in time!

OOOOOW! I SQUISHED MY VAJEEN!

Having fun yet? V-straddle injuries can happen because of bike riding, horseback riding, zip-lining, spinning, falling flat on your V, too-intense use of sex toys, and consensual over-the-top rough sex. Hematomas (collections of blood), bruises, and significant lacerations—or worse—can happen. Most of these injuries, if they're not more serious, are treated with TLC that includes ice packs for 24 hours, compression, rest, and sitz baths (see page 38). If you've really done a number on your who-ha, an examination under anesthesia, stitches, or more extensive surgical repair may be needed. Sure, less serious vulvar and vaginal cuts and bruises can be frightening because they bleed a lot. And vulvar hematomas are scary because some can expand to grapefruit size or even bigger. But no worries: Believe it or not, most will resolve spontaneously. In a rare case, your doctor may have to drain a hematoma with surgery, but even that will turn out a-OK.

A LAST WORD ABOUT WET WORKOUT CLOTHES Damp (or wet) swimsuits, gym clothes, yoga, Pilates, biking, spinning and running wear—all increase the chance for the growth of vaginal yeast and bacterial infections (BV). These bugs love moist, dark places. If you're prone to these conditions, don't hesitate. Change to dry clothing ASAP.

MORE HELPFUL HINTS FOR HAPPY TRAILS

- Use a wider seat.

- Don't tilt your seat upward; it could increase pressure on the vulva.

- Be sure your seat is at the correct height so that your legs aren't completely extended at the bottom of your pedal stroke.

- Raise the handlebars to help you sit more upright.

- Change your sitting position, and take breaks during long rides.

- If you experience tingling or numbness, get off your bike.

- Switch to a recumbent bike.

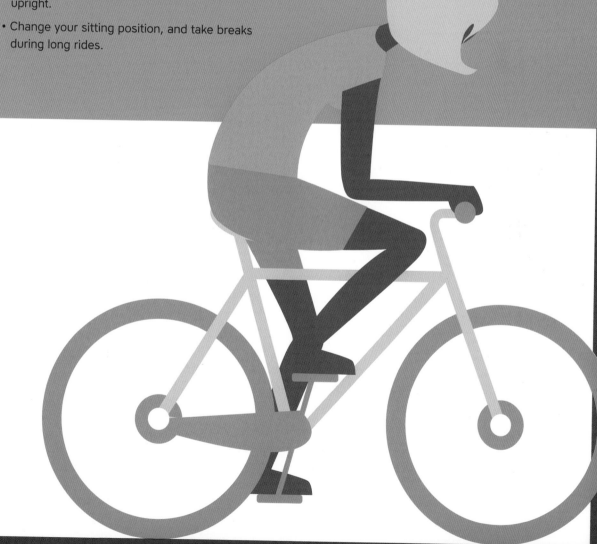

L

IS FOR LABIOPLASTY

Vaginoplasty and Other
Procedures for V-Vanity

There's a brave new world of designer vaginas: the latest trend in cosmetic surgery. People have been nipping, tucking, implanting, and vacuuming lots of body parts, and now some sisters are turning their quest for perfection to their genitals. Elective surgeries that promise a better sex life or more aesthetically pleasing private parts are gaining popularity at a gallop. But both the medical community and cultural busybodies are divided over whether these are valid, beneficial surgeries or just over-the-top who-ha obsessions. You decide.

HELP! I HATE MY LABIA. IT LOOKS FAT! CAN I PUT IT ON A DIET?

Sorry. Eliminating fried foods and gummy bears from your daily diet won't do it. But you're not alone in thinking your labia is chubby. More women than ever before are coming into my office worried their labia are too fat, too big, too floppy, uneven, wrinkly, saggy, or otherwise unsightly. Whether it's a misguided judgment call or the real deal is relative. First things first: Compassion and empathy are in order.

FYI The New View Campaign based in New York City is a feminist organization of social scientists and clinicians who oppose labioplasty. They claim these procedures are turning healthy female sexuality into a medical problem, thereby endangering women's health just for profit.

Labia shapes and sizes are remarkably variable, and there really is no "normal." But if you want to get technical, the typical labia minora is about 1 to 2 inches (3 to 4 cm) in width when held taught.

It's not wholly about L-looks. Women with larger ones can suffer from chronic irritation, infection, poor hygiene, and pain during sex or sports because of their floppy labia. It's true! Girls come to my office asking me to "fix my camel toe—please." And there's the emotional and psychological stress too. Some women just don't feel "beautiful or feminine enough down there." This is particularly heartbreaking in vulnerable teens too embarrassed to change in the locker room. Sometimes counseling and education about personal hygiene and clothing choices helps overcome the anxiety and dissatisfaction. But an increasing number of women are opting for surgery.

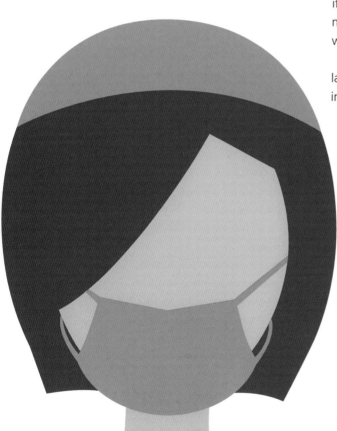

LABIOPLASTY

The vast majority of complaints involve the labia minora, and this cosmetic procedure reduces the dimensions of labia minora (inner part of the lips) or the labia majora (outer lips). Complications are rare but can include infection, bleeding, scarring, pigment changes, painful sex, or other poor cosmetic results. Less commonly, if the labia majora are "bulky and bulging," surgical revision and removal of fatty tissue and/or liposuction is an option. In other cases, when women complain of a "sagging and wrinkly" labia majora (because of things like advancing age, childbirth, or massive weight loss), collagen injections or autologous fat transplant (donation of fat from another area on your own body) may be the way to go. Laser treatments that create new collagen and more youthful-looking tissue are another avenue to explore. Laser vaginal and vulvar rejuvenation is not FDA approved at present but is gaining popularity.

Choosing surgery of any kind for these issues requires careful consideration, as does picking a gynecologic or plastic surgeon comfortable and experienced in genital rejuvenation procedures. Make finding a great doc a priority!

BOTOX WORKED WONDERS ON MY FOREHEAD WRINKLES. WHAT ABOUT ON MY LABIA?

Right now there's no cosmetic procedure for genitals that uses Botox injections. It is currently only used on genitals to treat extreme cases of vulvodynia (see page 86), and it may prove helpful down the road to alleviate other vulvar pain syndromes.

MY FRIEND JUST HAD A VAGINOPLASTY AND IS GUSHING OVER HER NEW QUIM. WHAT'S THE DEAL?

Whatever you call it, *vaginoplasty*, *designer vaginoplasty*, *vaginal rejuvenation*, or *revirgination*, they are, for the most part, variations on traditional vaginal surgical procedures. When combined with labioplasty, these operations promise to make your vajayjay tighter, narrower, and more youthful and ultra-sensitive. While the surgeon is at it, bulges of your bladder, rectum, or vagina can be tucked away, and the hymen can be repaired and remodeled.

These procedures may be medically suggested for some women with vaginal-wall relaxation or bulging and hanging genital organs. But plenty of women are pursuing the treatment for the sole purpose of beautification and improved personal and partner sexual satisfaction. Surgery purely for cosmetic reason and sexual enhancement should be approached intelligently and pursued with an experienced provider.

> *I see my body as an instrument, rather than an ornament.*
>
> —Alanis Morissette, Quoted in
> *Reader's Digest*

EVER SINCE I GAVE BIRTH, THE SPACE BETWEEN MY V AND RECTUM IS SAGGING. IS THERE ANYTHING I CAN DO ABOUT IT?

Yes, there's a procedure called perineoplasty, which tightens that area. It promises to lend a more youthful appearance to the vulva and a tighter vaginal opening for enhanced sexual function.

MY PUBIC AREA IS HUMONGOUS. CAN ANYTHING BE DONE WITH IT?

Are you talking about the mons pubis, the fleshy mound of fat over your pubic bone? True, the mons pubis can get flabby or saggy particularly with age or weight gain, and some women feel theirs is too bulky and unsightly and can be seen through their swimsuit or gym clothes. There are treatments available to reduce the size of the mons pubis, including liposuction and contouring.

OMG! G-SPOT AMPLIFICATION

Want to enhance your sexual satisfaction? Some women choose to do it by making their G-spot bigger. Amplification typically involves an injection of collagen (the main structural protein found in animal connective tissue—the "glue" that helps hold the body together and gives our skin strength and elasticity) into the anterior wall of the vagina. Warning: There is no scientific information on the safety, efficacy, or long-term satisfaction of this procedure. A doc can also perform an O-Shot procedure in which they inject the clitoris with autologous plasma cells (plasma cells separated out of your own blood and reinjected where you want "new growth," in this case, the clit) with the intention of enhancing orgasm and improving sexual function. You should also investigate your concerns about sexual satisfaction and/or sexual dysfunction with your gyno or therapist. Ladies, don't make this decision lightly.

FIRST AND FOREMOST—RESEARCH, DISCUSS, AND PONDER Choosing surgery of any kind for aesthetic or pleasure issues requires careful consideration, as does choosing a gynecologic or plastic surgeon who is comfortable and experienced in genital rejuvenation procedures. Do not proceed unless you've done your homework!

If men could menstruate . . . clearly, menstruation would become an enviable, boast-worthy, masculine event: Men would brag about how long and how much. . . . Sanitary supplies would be federally funded and free.

—Gloria Steinem

I'VE HEARD ABOUT VAGINAL REJUVENATION SPAS. ARE THEY FOR REAL?

Yup! They're popping up all over the place in DC, NYC, LA, Palm Beach, Phoenix, even San Miguel, Mexico! These so-called vagina spas promise to turn your already naturally fantastic V into an organ of extraordinary beauty and vitality worthy of a diamond tiara. Special exercises to improve pelvic muscle tone, which helps with bladder control as well as orgasm enhancement, are offered with names like Kegel Phitness, the "Other" Face Lift, and Lip Sync. Many spas offer a full range of vaginal cosmetic surgery or liposuction techniques. You can get your vagina massaged or have one-on-one vaginal exercise instruction. There's also Gwyneth Paltrow's choice: herbal steaming for the V. Supposedly this procedure enhances vulvar and vaginal health, soothes PMS, and even improves fertility. The practice is done in fancy spas or you can even DIY, but its effects are controversial at best. Done absolutely correctly, it can be warm and relaxing and bring blood flow to the area. Done incorrectly, it's not pretty: Irritation, burns, infections, and more can occur.

Another treatment is Linger—an "internal feminine flavoring" treatment that promises to keep your vagina in mint condition. Think of it as an Altoids for your lady parts.

COMMON COMPLAINTS FROM THE OWNERS OF LARGER LABIAS

- I hate wearing a swimsuit or anything spandex like yoga pants because it looks like there's a pillow between my legs.

- I have to fold up my labia and push it into my vagina so the bulge isn't huge.

- Nothing slips into my vagina easily— especially tampons and penises. Why? Because of these big lips!

M

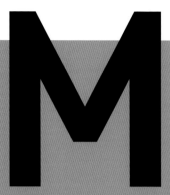

IS FOR MENSTRUATION, MOODS, AND MISERY

Everything You Need to Know
to Make It Through

Aunt Flow, Cousin Red, the Present or Gift or
Visitor, Get (one's) redwings, have the painters
in, on the rag, red tide, ride the cotton pony,
Sally, surf the crimson wave, that time of
the month, your period . . . Listen, whatever
you want to call it—you've got it. You're
menstruating.

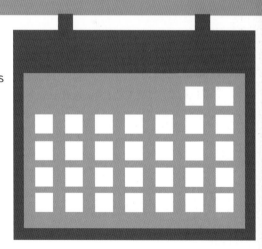

WHAT EXACTLY HAPPENS WHEN I GET MY PERIOD?

It's this simple: When you menstruate—or get your period—your body sheds the lining of the uterus (womb). Menstrual blood flows from the uterus through the small opening in your cervix and passes out of your body through the vajayjay. And sometimes, or even usually, it's not much fun.

HOW LONG DOES A NORMAL PERIOD LAST?

Most menstrual periods last from 3 to 7 days. The average menstrual cycle lasts 28 to 30 days counting from the first day of one period to the first day of the next, but normal cycles can vary from 21 to 45 days. During an average menses, women lose approximately 5 tablespoons, up to 80 milliliters, of blood—though it often seems like a lot more than that! There is a ton of variation in what's considered normal, but in general if you are using more than six to ten pads or tampons per day or soaking through one to two super pads or tampons every hour, let your doctor know, as this is more than the norm and you might have an issue like uterine fibroids, polyps, or, on rare occasions, cancer. Also, if you always wear a yellow polka dot skirt with chartreuse striped halter top every day when you have your period and insist on putting petunias in your hair, I'd say that's probably not normal either. See your mirror.

AT WHAT AGE DOES THE RED TIDE USUALLY START?

Well, it can begin as early as 8 years old or as late as 16. Most often it begins between 11 and 12 years. FYI: The start of menstruation has its own name: menarche. Sounds French, *oui*? Young femmes should not freak if their menstruation cycle is irregular—it takes a while to get into a rhythm.

I DON'T GET MY PERIOD EVERY MONTH, BUT WHEN IT COMES ... OMG ... IT'S IMPRESSIVE. HOW WEIRD IS THAT?

Well, it's not that weird. There are a few reasons this could be happening, and you should get checked out. It's common in adolescents and perimenopausal women or those with PCOS (polycystic ovarian syndrome). Also, an abnormal growth in the uterus can lead to "weird" menses. This includes uterine polyps (fleshy growths, typically benign), fibroids (benign muscular tumors), hyperplasia (an overgrowth of uterine tissue and possible cancer precursor), and uterine cancer. Finally, a bleeding disorder such as Von Willebrand disease (a clotting disorder) or a low platelet count (these are blood cells that help blood to clot) can cause a heavy flow. Blood thinning medications such as Coumadin or aspirin may also cause abnormal periods. Don't wait around—see your doc.

TALKING THE TALK

Sisters, we know how "special" we feel when we have our periods (ha-ha)— maybe that's why menstruation has so many special words to define its many manifestations. Here they are:

MENORRHAGIA The medical term for heavy or prolonged menstrual bleeding.

METRORRHAGIA Bleeding between periods.

POLYMENORRHEA Frequent menstrual bleeding, specifically, bleeding that occurs every 21 days or more frequently.

AMENORRHEA The absence of menses. Primary amenorrhea is when your period hasn't started by age 16, secondary amenorrhea is when menses are absent for more than three to six months, and . . .

OLIGOMENORRHEA Fewer than six to eight periods per year.

ANOVULATION When you don't ovulate. Yea, you say, if you're not looking to get on the baby carriage trail? Well, it can also mean you end up with a heavy period or menses when you do.

FYI: If you have any of these conditions, see your doctor!

GOT CRAMPS? Have sex! Orgasms can relieve menstrual cramps in some women.

MY CRAMPS ARE NO JOKE!

Does it help to know you're not alone? Probably not much. But let me tell you, menstrual cramps of some degree affect more than 50 percent of us, and up to 15 percent of women describe their menstrual cramps as way severe. Surveys of adolescent girls show that over 90 percent report having menstrual cramps. They can range from mild to quite severe. Mild menstrual cramps may be barely noticeable and of short duration—sometimes it's just a slight sense of heaviness in the belly. Severe menstrual cramps can be so painful that they interfere with a woman's regular activities for several days. If this is you—let your doctor know about it.

HOW TO TREAT THOSE CRAMPS

- Use a heating pad.

- Think ahead and take NSAIDs (such as Advil) a day or so before your period.

- Ask your gyno about hormonal contraception.

- Get treatment for any underlying condition causing the cramps.

Q. How did the Red Sea get its name?
A. Cleopatra used to bathe there periodically.

RIGHT BEFORE MY PERIOD I'M A BITCH ON WHEELS!

And let me guess: Your partner is the pavement. The physical and emotional changes that happen during the days before you get your period are called PMS, premenstrual syndrome. PMS affects at least 85 percent of menstruating women and the symptoms are physical and emotional, but guess what? (and don't get annoyed) the cause is unknown. PMDD, premenstrual dysphoric disorder, is a severe form of PMS that affects a small percentage of women, in which symptoms interfere substantially with work or personal relationships. Does that sound like you? Get help.

FROM THE AWESOME-JOKE FILES

The ten definitive signs of PMS are:

1. You feel like every soul you know took an obnoxious pill.
2. You love to put tortilla chips in your mint ice cream and think Cheetos are the bomb.
3. Your friends, family, and partner are cowering in the corner—for good reason.
4. You've got a serious case of f'n potty mouth.
5. Your waiter is the most annoying person on earth. Make that everyone within two feet.
6. You want seconds—and where's the dessert?
7. You're looking forward to menopause.
8. You're can't avoid bumping into people and things and blame everything and everyone for getting in your way.
9. You really hate men.
10. You want sex. You don't want sex. You want sex. You don't want sex. You want sex . . .

IS THERE ANY WAY I CAN STOP FEELING SO CRAZY?

Absolutely!

- Try regular aerobic exercise, relaxation through yoga, meditation, breathing exercises, and getting enough sleep. Okay, maybe you don't have time for all of these, but the more you do, the better off you'll be.

- Make some dietary changes. Dishes rich in complex carbohydrates can reduce mood symptoms and food cravings. Avoiding caffeine and alcohol may help, but so may that glass of wine. Drink in moderation if it lifts your spirit, but avoid it if it just compounds your moodiness. Eat less fat, salt, and sugar, and eating small, frequent meals is also a good idea.

- Use supplements during the height of your symptoms. Taking 1,200 mg of calcium a day at this time can reduce PMS symptoms. Magnesium may help reduce water retention, breast tenderness, headaches, and mood symptoms. The B vitamins, especially when you get them from your diet (good sources are fortified cereals, beans, dark leafy greens, fish, papayas, cantaloupe, and oranges), can also help relieve symptoms.

- Check with your doctor about prescription meds. For those who really go off the PMS deep end, hormonal contraceptives like the pill may lessen the physical symptoms. Low-dose diuretics, or water pills, can help with water retention. Finally, certain antidepressants can be used, typically on days 14 to 28 of the cycle or every day if need be. Antianxiety pills may also be right for some sisters.

THE SCOOP ON SANITARY PRODUCTS

PADS These come in different sizes, styles, and thicknesses. Some have wings that fold under your underwear for better protection. Some are fragrant; avoid these if they irritate your skin.

PANTY LINERS Thinner and shorter than pads, liners are for lighter flow and come in various shapes and sizes, including those meant for thongs.

TAMPONS Available in a variety of sizes depending on flow, tampons can be fragranced, and come with or without an applicator. They should not be left in for more than eight hours and usually need to be changed more frequently. Tampons can be worn while swimming and exercising without a prob.

NOTE: For the supersensitive or environmentally conscious, there are organic and all-cotton varieties of pads, liners, and tampons. You can even sign up for a monthly mail-order delivery of these products.

MENSTRUAL CUP (AKA DIVACUP) This nonabsorbent soft silicone reusable cup is inserted into the vagina and collects menstrual flow. It can be worn for up to 12 hours and eliminates the need for other sanitary products as it acts as a barrier.

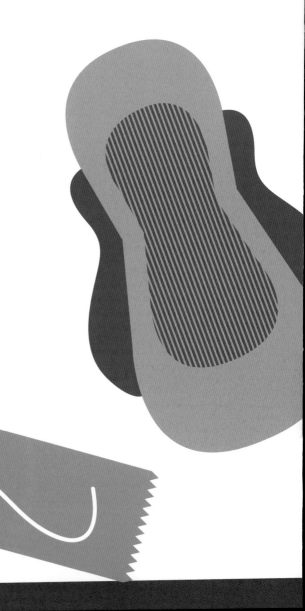

PMS SYMPTOMS (AS IF I HAVE TO TELL YOU)

EMOTIONAL SYMPTOMS depression, angry outbursts, irritability, crying spells, anxiety, confusion, social withdrawal, poor concentration, insomnia, increased nap taking, changes in sexual desire

PHYSICAL SYMPTOMS thirst and appetite changes including food cravings, breast tenderness, bloating and weight gain, headache, swelling of the hands or feet, aches and pains, fatigue, skin problems, gastrointestinal symptoms, abdominal pain

NOTE: Symptoms of other common conditions can mimic or overlap with PMS, such as depression and anxiety, perimenopause, chronic fatigue syndrome, irritable bowel syndrome, and thyroid disease to name a few. In addition, certain conditions may worsen right before your period such as seizure disorders, migraines, asthma, and allergies.

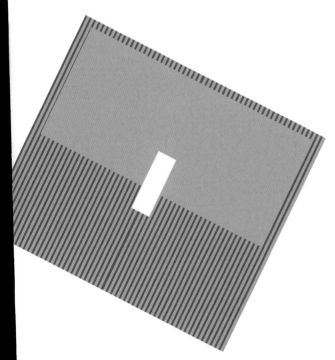

MENSTRUAL SPONGE Literally a sponge from the sea, it comes in various levels of absorbency. A sponge is inserted into the vagina to absorb the blood, then rinsed out and used again. This sounds great, but sponges haven't been FDA approved or rigorously studied for safety. They can cause infection and allergic reactions, and possibly dissolve inside the vagina and be absorbed by the body. As with tampons, there is also the potential of toxic shock syndrome (TSS).

REUSABLE MENSTRUAL PADS These are exactly what they sound like, and for the environmentally obsessed who don't mind getting very up close and personal with their menses, these typically cloth pads are an awesome option.

N

IS FOR NUTRITION

A Guide to Know-How
and No-No's for Your Lady-
Parts-Related Health

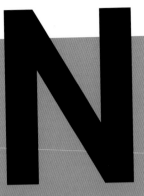

YOU KNOW THE OLD SAYING "YOU ARE WHAT YOU EAT"? WHAT SHOULD I EAT TO KEEP MY VAG SWEET AND HEALTHY?

The answer is not sugar, honey. The fact is any diet that is healthy for your entire body will benefit your V. But if your vagina isn't getting the balance of vitamins and minerals it needs, you could be more prone to irritation and infection, making for one unhappy vajayjay.

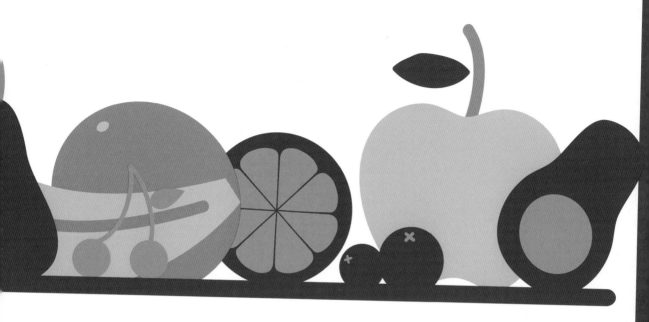

MY GYNECOLOGIST TOLD ME TO TAKE CALCIUM AND VITAMIN D, BUT I'M NOT CLEAR WHY.

First of all, sister, if you don't understand something your doc tells you, ask questions. Vitamin D and calcium are usually suggested for bone health—and the vagina is boneless, so it makes sense that you're confused. BUT these supplements have other benefits, too. The Institute of Medicine, which is an independent, nonprofit organization, recommends for overall good health a total daily calcium intake of 1,300 mg for girls aged 9 to 18, 1,000 mg for women aged 19 to 50, and 1,200 mg for women 51 and older. And, as said before, if you want a healthy vagina, you need a healthy body. While it's best to get your calcium in foods such as dairy, broccoli, almonds, and salmon, supplements may also be needed. Calcium supplements should be taken in divided doses. Don't take more than 600 mg at a time because your body will have a tougher time absorbing it. And don't overdo! Too much calcium can lead to kidney stones.

So, what about vitamin D? You need it to absorb the calcium. Fortified dairy products provide dietary D, but the main source is sunlight. Since most of us slather ourselves with sunscreen—and you should—supplemental vitamin D of 1,000 IU/day or less is a safe alternative.

WHAT TO EAT

- Yogurt—the key ingredient, live cultures, is a huge help in preventing and treating yeast infections. You can also take acidophilus supplements.

- Fruits, vegetables, whole grains, which promote overall good health.

- Cranberry juice or supplements, which decrease the chance of a urinary tract infection in those who are prone to them.

WHAT TO AVOID

- Foods high in sugar have a tendency to increase the risk of yeast infections. Processed foods, baked goods, alcohol, and sweet drinks should be avoided for the same reason.

ALERT! Eating disorders such as anorexia, bulimia, and the college-popular orthorexia (obsession with only eating foods one considers healthy) or drunkorexia (a slang term for the real problem of self-starvation or binging/purging as a means of weight control for planned binge drinking) can cause menstrual irregularity or even amenorrhea. Prolonged amenorrhea is linked to low bone mass and then osteoporosis.

Don't eat anything your great-great grandmother wouldn't recognize as food. There are a great many food-like items in the supermarket your ancestors wouldn't recognize as food.

—Michael Pollan

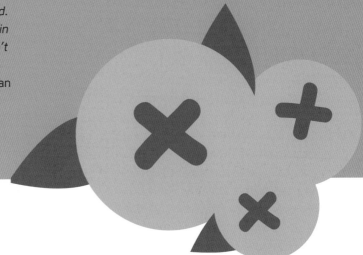

Good sex is like a good bridge game. If you don't have a good partner, you'd better have a good hand.

—Mae West

WANNA FEEL SEXY? LOVE YOUR BODY!

A common cause of low sex drive in women is poor body image. A healthy diet and regular exercise are the keys to helping you feel like a red-hot mama. Regular exercise also increases blood flow to the genitals and increases the body's production of endorphins, those "feel good" chemicals.

ARE THERE ANY NATURAL HERBS THAT CAN GIVE MY SEX DRIVE A BOOST?

There are no guarantees, but you can try arginine, which is an amino acid found in granola, oatmeal, nuts, seeds, eggs, coconut milk, and root veggies, or you can get it in a supplement form. It claims to increase blood flow to the genitals and enhance sex drive.

WHAT ABOUT APHRODISIACS?

- Chocolate contains phenylethylamine and serotonin, chemicals that promote a feeling of well-being.

- Red wine is relaxing and contains resveratrol, an antioxidant that helps boost blood flow and improve circulation.

- Oysters contain zinc, which enhances sexual potency in men, and omega-3 fatty acids, which improve nervous system functions.

- Bananas have a suggestive phallic shape and contain potassium, which promotes strong muscles.

- Avocado (note its phallic "testicular" shape) contains vitamin E, which is helpful in hormonal production and thus sexual response.

- Salmon and walnuts contain omega-3 fatty acids needed for the production of sex hormones (estrogen, progesterone, testosterone).

- Chili peppers contain capsaicin, which causes sweating and increases heart rate and circulation—even in the genitals!

- Figs are sexually suggestive based on appearance, since they look similar to sex organs.

- Honey is rich in B vitamins and boron, needed for the production of sex hormones (mainly testosterone).

- Soy in the diet and in supplement form contains isoflavones, which promote vaginal lubrication due to their estrogen-like qualities (high-volume intake may not be appropriate for women with breast cancer).

ALERT Keep in mind that excess amounts of some vitamins or minerals, and many herbal supplements, can be harmful during pregnancy. Speak with your doc before taking any.

- Folic acid (folate) lowers the risk of neural tube defects such as spina bifida.

- Iron will help prevent anemia, or a low count of red blood cells, or hemoglobin in the blood.

- Omega-3 fatty acids (aka DHA), found in many fish, help promote a healthy nervous system.

I'M PREGNANT. SHOULD I TAKE SPECIAL VITAMINS?

Prenatal vitamins are recommended for most women during pregnancy in order to obtain the extra recommended daily intake (RDI) of omega-3 fatty acids, iron, and folic acid. Here's why you need those things:

WHAT ABOUT GAINING WEIGHT WHILE I'M PREGNANT?

Well, you don't want to go overboard, but you should definitely pack on some pounds. Most moms-to-be who are already a healthy weight should gain between 25 and 35 pounds (11 and 16 kg) during pregnancy. An additional 300 calories a day is a good rule, and small, frequent meals rather than three large ones are often best. But like most things in life, it's best not to overdo it. Keep in mind: Excessive weight gain increases the risk for gestational diabetes and/or very big babies. That means a tough delivery and the possibility of more extensive V-trauma.

O

IS FOR ORGASMS!

The Big O! Oh! Oh! Oh!
Ahhh . . . All Things Orgasmic
and Otherwise

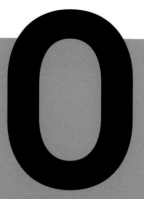

Sure, like this is news: Unlike guys, we need to be in the mood to have sex. If we're stressed, pissed off, feeling fat or unattractive, slightly short of smelling like a rose or not totally groomed, thinking about the laundry, angsting over our kids, worried about work, down and blue, freaked out about exams, exhausted, achy, not feeling safe, or dealing with money woes, the chance we're going to feel like hot babes and have an orgasm is pretty low. Plus, there are plenty of ways to get physical and emotional comfort without intercourse or orgasm. So, even though some of us can take the oh oh oh or leave it—and other sisters may be in it just to please their partners—lots of us want and need the BIG O and we'll do whatever to have one. Wait! Make that two or three.

I KNOW WHAT IT FEELS LIKE. BUT I'M CURIOUS ABOUT WHAT'S HAPPENING TO MY BODY WHILE I'M COMING.

We call the desire to have sex the libido. Your libido can suddenly be charged up for no apparent reason, or because your partner is making you hot, or because other thoughts or images are turning you on.

Arousal, on the other hand, is the result of sexual stimulation plus desire. Your body knows it: Your blood pressure, heart rate, breathing rate, and body temperature all rise. Your nips are erect, and your labia and clit are engorged with blood and supersensitive. Your cha cha is juicy and expands. It's sayin' "Come and get me!" Well, hold on . . . you're almost there. Contractions of the genital muscles and then . . . and then . . . an overwhelming feeling of release. Mmmmmm . . . . that was intense.

FACTOID Orgasms can cause bad breath! Doctors have detected a slight odor on the tongues of women for up to an hour after they've had intercourse. Note to self: Keep some gum or mints on the nightstand.

I USED TO BE HOT; I REALLY LOVE SEX AND WAS THE REIGNING QUEEN OF O. NOW IT TAKES FOREVER OR WORSE, IT DOESN'T HAPPEN AT ALL. AND HONESTLY, I COULDN'T CARE LESS.

It probably doesn't make you feel any better to know probs in this department aren't uncommon. And there usually isn't just one reason keeping you from wanting to have sex or reaching a climax. Best advice? Be open about it and speak with your gyno. I can promise this issue is raised over and over again. Join in the discussion. Meanwhile, here are a few possibilities:

GETTING OLDER You might still look as hot as Jennifer Lopez, but your libido doesn't know it and it slows down as the years add up. Usually this is not a five alarmer unless it's interfering with your relationship. Declining estrogen and androgens (male hormones) because of aging or natural or surgical menopause may lessen your desire for sex.

ONE OF THE BIG SHOCKS of the twentieth century was that our nation's sex symbol, Marilyn Monroe, claimed she never achieved orgasm by any of her famous lovers (John F. Kennedy, Frank Sinatra, Joe DiMaggio, etc.).

Electric flesh-arrows traversing the body; a rainbow of color strikes the eyelids. A foam of music falls over the ears. It is the gong of the orgasm.

—Anaïs Nin

MEDICATIONS Occasionally, medications such as birth control pills, SSRI antidepressants, and beta-blockers used to treat high blood pressure can alter libido.

MEDICAL ISSUES Coronary artery disease, arthritis, cancer, diabetes, and other conditions may affect your sex drive. Depression is a very common cause of decreased libido. In fact, sometimes it's hard to know whether decreased desire is because you're feeling down—or taking medications to beat it—or a combo of both. Total bummer.

BODY IMAGE The way you think and feel about yourself plays a huge role in sexual desire. Sisters who feel unattractive, overweight, or out of shape are more likely to avoid sex altogether.

FYI Some women scream, some women moan, some women whimper, some women LOL, some women weep, some women thank God, some women recite Emily Dickinson, some women curse, some women stay silent.

RELATIONSHIP PROBLEMS These can definitely put a damper on sex. That's why desire is so much more intense and sex is more frequent when you're with a new partner—you don't have any problems to dwell on yet—and libido can become dulled and sex less frequent in long-term relationships. This is only a problem if you or your partner is unhappy about having less nookie. BUT if you can't get turned on because you resent your partner, well, that's another story and a marriage counselor or therapist might be in order.

SMOKING, ALCOHOL, DRUGS Bad habits like these can definitely lower your sex drive and response. Smoking in particular decreases the blood flow to the genitals and can cause issues with arousal. Ladies, another reason to quit! And when it comes to alcohol, small amounts might decrease inhibitions and enhance sexual drive, but too much drink is a depressant and often has the opposite effect.

DEALING WITH IT

So, if you want to hop back on the saddle, you've got to discover and then deal with the underlying issues. To get back on the road to O (or travel it more frequently):

- Set up a time to talk to your partner about it.

- Diet, exercise, and a healthy lifestyle are key.

- Stress reduction and adequate sleep are essential.

- Be sure you're setting aside time for intimacy without other distractions. Shut off the television, computer, cell phone; be sure the kids are asleep or your roommate is not going to walk in. Here's a suggestion: Put a lock on the door! Amazing what this small effort can do for the libido. There's no worse buzzkill than the threat of someone, especially kids, bursting into the room.

- Consider over-the-counter (OTC) supplements although effectiveness is varied. Supplements containing arginine promise increased desire and pleasure. Zestra, a botanical massage oil, which claims to increase arousal, can be applied to the clitoris, labia, and vagina. DHEA is an OTC nutritional supplement and a chemical precursor to testosterone. Warning: Though some of these products are FDA cleared as nutritional supplements, they are not held to the same rigorous standard as FDA-approved drugs.

TOO BAD Medications prescribed for men, like Viagra and Cialis, are not on the list of approved drugs for women . . . yet.

- Try testosterone therapy, which is available by prescription. It's been proven to improve sexual function in many women and is often used "off label" for this purpose (meaning it is prescribed for an issue other than its stated purpose). But check this out: There are potential side effects to consider including deepening of the voice, acne, hair growth in typically male places (upper lip, chin), enlarged clitoris, and alteration in lipid profile.

WHAT ABOUT ADDYI?

Addyi is a newly approved med for the 10 percent of women suffering with HSDD (hypoactive sexual desire disorder, a dysfunction that causes a severely decreased to nonexistent sex drive, causing distress). Although Addyi is often referred to as the "female Viagra," that's not quite right. Viagra and similar meds increase blood flow to the penis to correct a mechanical problem with the erection. On the contrary, Addyi works in the brain. It's taken daily rather than on demand and can cause sleepiness and low blood pressure. It's currently indicated for premenopausal women only. If you take it, you should avoid alcohol.

Other meds are on the horizon to help with female sexual desire, so stay tuned!

> *Memory is like an orgasm. It's a lot better if you don't have to fake it.*
>
> —Anonymous

WANNA HAVE AN ORGASM? WELL . . .

It's not always about the penis. Some of us won't have an orgasm with vaginal intercourse alone but can come with manual clitoral stimulation from a partner, a vibrator, or masturbation. There are lots of vibrators on the market that vary in price and can definitely do the trick. There's also a new kid on the block called Fiera, a sleek and discreet device that attaches to the clitoris to improve arousal and potentially enhance an orgasm by boosting clitoral blood flow.

IT'S JUST NOT HAPPENING, AND I'M MISERABLE. I TRIED PRACTICALLY EVERYTHING. WHAT ELSE CAN I DO?

Has anyone spoken to you about sex therapy? You can either go alone or with your partner to a specially trained physician, psychologist, or social worker. Usually the therapy session will include education about the normal sexual response, as well as ways to deal with cultural, religious, and personal sexual concerns. Sex therapists work to improve communication and enhance trust and intimacy between partners. They use visual aids, devices, and give "homework." Therapy may help partners agree on sexual practices and frequency. Visit www.aasect.org for further information.

NOTE: Ladies with prior sexual, emotional, or physical abuse often benefit from collaboration with a trained mental health professional. Those with an underlying medical condition causing sexual problems would benefit from an appropriate physician referral as well. A team approach is best in these cases.

As many as two-thirds of women admit to faking orgasms at some point in their lives—and it's not just during vaginal intercourse. Women also say they have pretended to orgasm during oral and phone sex. Remember when Harry met Sally?

FAKING IT

Well, lots of my patients fake it and admit to it, and it's no big deal. Although there may be a twinge of guilt, they have their reasons: they want to please their partner, they feel "sorry" for their partner and don't want to cause any embarrassment or feelings of inadequacy, or they just want to get it over with so they can get some sleep. As long as a woman can have an orgasm, it's no biggie if there's no O every time she makes love. Sometimes a gal's gotta do what a gal's gotta do.

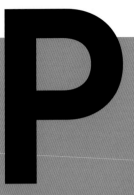

P

IS FOR PERSONAL HYGIENE

The Dirty Secret about Douches,
Soaps, Perfumes, and Our Obsession
to Be Wiped Out

Gawd. After watching countless TV commercials, looking at endless glossy magazine and online ads, you'd think our vaginas are filthy places in desperate need of top-to-bottom cleaning. Ha! That's a big fat V lie. The truth is that our bodies naturally possess a delicate balance of yeast and bacteria aimed at keeping our vaginas in tip-top condition. It's awesome. But is that good enough for those advertising dudes who want to spread the silly word that we need to buy products in order for our coochies to smell sweet? Nah. It's bogus because too much "cleaning" and seemingly helpful "hygiene" products can actually cause itching, irritation, even infection by disrupting our natural balance of bacteria. Sisters, please listen:

My vagina doesn't need to be cleaned up. It smells good already. Don't try to decorate.

—Eve Ensler,
The Vagina Monologues

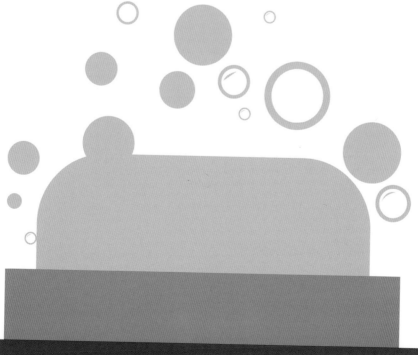

Your vagina does its own cleaning by naturally keeping pH levels in a delicate balance, though this can be disrupted by using antibiotics, douches, harsh soaps, and other products that may cause irritation or infection. That said, the smell of your vagina is directly related to your health, lifestyle, weight, and diet. Remember, some vaginal discharge is normal—while foul odor, copious discharge, itching, and irritation are messages to get prompt medical attention.

SAVE YOUR MONEY AND YOUR VAJAYJAY

SOAPS There are some lovely ladies who can use any product on their vag and it's cool, no problemo. But if you have sensitive skin or you're suffering from vulvar or vaginal dryness, you might want to ditch the harsh or highly fragrant soap and consider using a mild soap such as Ivory or Dove or a moisturizing wash such as Lubrigyn. Remember, the inside of your V itself doesn't need to be vigorously scrubbed. Some ladies find it helpful to use soap only on the vulva and use plain warm water on the more delicate vaginal mucous membranes. Vigorous scrubbing with a washcloth or abrasive sponge, particularly inside the vagina, should be avoided. When taking a bath, dilute pure oils, such as lavender, with just a few drops in the tub, since they can also be highly irritating.

FRAGRANCES/PERFUMES AND FOUL ODORS Women, it's a fact: The vagina typically has a sweet smell. Under normal circumstances, or even if you have an infection, it's likely that no one else notices an odor from your vagina (except maybe your sex partner). Regarding your period, if you change pads or tampons frequently enough and bathe regularly, no one can smell that either. Feminine sprays,

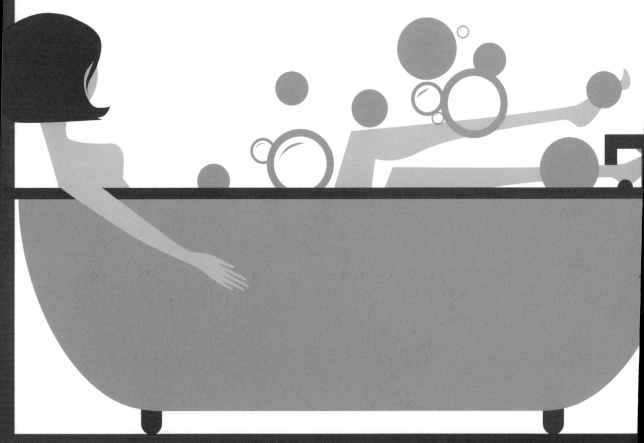

deodorants, and scented tampons are heavily perfumed and can lead to allergic reactions, irritation, and infection. Avoid these. If you have sensitive skin, use a fragrance-free laundry detergent and fabric softener on your undergarments and opt for dye-free TP.

POWDER/TALC/BABY WIPES Hey, baby, guess what? You're a grown woman, so ditch the baby products. Don't use powders that contain talc at any age, as it may be associated with an increased risk of ovarian cancer. (Read about talc's association with ovarian cancer on page 124.) Cornstarch and talc-free baby powders are safe to sprinkle in your underwear or directly on your vulva and skin to prevent chafing and perspiration, but baby wipes can be very irritating for sensitive V's.

DOUCHING The vagina cleanses itself and that's why douching should probably be avoided altogether. This silly product-driven practice can disturb the natural balance of vaginal organisms; altering your vaginal pH can actually cause pelvic infection. Douching after your period, in fact, can push blood and bacteria into the pelvis. So . . . *DON'T DOUCHE!*

I DON'T USE ANY PRODUCTS, BUT MY LADY FLOWER IS STILL OFF-BALANCE.

That's because there are other everyday irritants:

PANTY HOSE/UNDERWEAR Yeast and bacteria love to live in moist, dark, non-aerated places. Wearing cotton underwear (or, at the very least, cotton crotched) and avoiding panty hose will allow for more airflow to your V and prevent infection and irritation. Better yet, go commando, especially at night.

PANTY LINERS/PADS Try to avoid these when you don't have your period since they allow for less airflow to the vagina and may promote infection and skin irritation. Fragrant pads are particularly problematic since they often cause skin reactions. (As an aside, some women I've seen come in because of irritation and a rash, and on exam, the outline of a pad is clearly depicted on the vulva like a drawing, making this the obvious source of the problem.) Constant contact with a wet or moist pad (designed for menstruation or urine leakage) can also cause the rash, so be sure to change your pad frequently.

SWIMSUITS/WORKOUT CLOTHES Try to get out of your wet swimsuit or workout clothes as soon as possible to avoid infection and irritation. Riding a bike or taking spinning classes increases the risk of chafing, so wear good padded shorts and consider a gel seat or moisture-barrier salve for better cushioning, especially for a lengthy class or long bicycle ride.

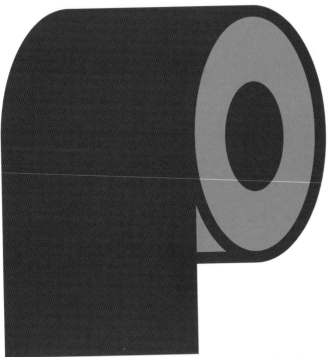

TIPS MADE SIMPLE

- Do keep your vulva clean and dry; if you are prone to infection or irritation, consider using a hair dryer on low/cool when coming out of the shower or tub.

- Don't wear tight-fitting pants or underwear; opt for cotton.

- Don't wear panty hose unless they have a cotton crotch; cut out the crotch if need be.

- Don't use pads or tampons that have deodorant or a plastic coating (not including the insertion tube or wrapper).

- Do use tampons only if you have your period, and choose a tampon that is only as absorbent as you need.

- Don't use perfumed soap or scented toilet paper.

- Don't douche or use feminine sprays or products containing talc.*

- Don't sleep in tight-fitting garments.

* In May 2016, a woman was granted $5 million in compensatory damages and $50 million in punitive damages from a lawsuit claiming Johnson & Johnson's talcum-powder–based products caused her ovarian cancer. This verdict adds to a continuing debate that is gathering momentum about the safety of talc-based cosmetic products. The verdict came just three months after Johnson & Johnson was ordered to pay $72 million in damages to the family of a different woman who also had died from ovarian cancer. Despite these two losses, the company still insists their products are safe. As of this writing, J&J plans to appeal the most recent decision.

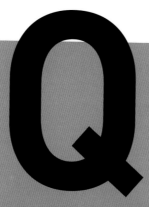

Q

IS FOR QUANDARIES

Abnormalities, Problems, Snafus, and the Complexities of Quims

Sisters, sometimes the vagina lets us down. Try as we do to keep it happy, there are conditions that perplex, vex, puzzle, mystify, bewilder, flummox, stupefy, dumbfound, and alas, make us blue. It's not pretty. That doesn't mean there aren't explanations and answers, but they may not solve the problem forever nor make us happy. In this chapter, we'll look at some of these situations. Just know that whatever you're going through, I have most likely seen it before—you're not alone. And remember:

NOTHING IS TOO GROSS TO TALK ABOUT.

The intimacy you share with your gyno can be similar to what you share with your hairdresser. A good gyno is a great listener. Plus, we never tell! That's the law.

What's the big mystery? It's my vagina, not the Sphinx!

—Miranda on
Sex and the City

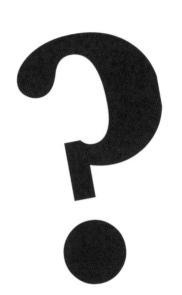

BARTHOLIN'S CYSTS/ABSCESSES

The Bartholin's glands are located at the opening of your V. If you're into exact locations, imagine your vajayjay is a clock and the gland ducts are located at the four and eight o'clock positions. If the opening of your gland becomes blocked, a cyst can develop. Don't freak out if this happens; it's not uncommon. Bartholin's cysts are usually between the size of a pea and a golf ball and can cause pain during sex or even when you're just walking or sitting. Obviously, it's no fun. If you're uncomfortable, your gyno will probably suggest draining the cyst. If it isn't bothering you, you can take a wait and see approach to see if it grows or becomes infected. If the cyst does get infected, you'll know it because it really hurts and draining will definitely be in order. Once it's drained of pus, the pain leaves immediately. The good news is that sometimes draining happens spontaneously while taking sitz baths or warm soaks. If not, you may need to have it done surgically. Also, antibiotics and pain medication may be prescribed. ***BUMMER ALERT: HISTORY CAN REPEAT ITSELF.***

VULVAR ABSCESS

This usually starts out as simple infection in the vulvar skin. What causes it? Risk factors include obesity, poor hygiene, and shaving or waxing. Sometimes a vulvar abscess will develop because your immune system isn't working well enough to fight infections. If your doc finds a tender, red, swollen, and painful collection of pus on your vulva, a diagnosis of a vulvar abscess will probably be made. Treatment includes antibiotics, drainage, warm soaks, and a follow-up to be sure the infection hasn't traveled beneath the skin level. ***BUMMER ALERT: IT CAN HAPPEN AGAIN.***

VAGINAL POLYPS AND CYSTS

Polyps are fleshy growths that are typically benign and won't need any treatment (yay!) unless they are growing, are painful, or cause bleeding. Cysts form when a gland or duct is clogged and liquid collects in a sac. These can occur inside the vagina. Again, treatment is not needed unless they are getting bigger or making you uncomfortable.

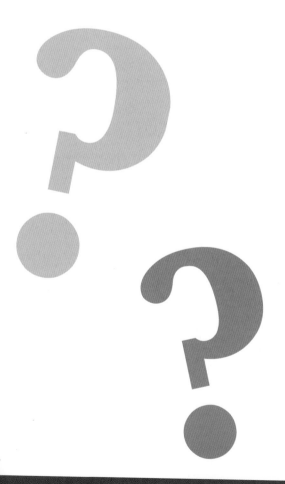

VULVAR SKIN TAGS

These are outgrowths of normal skin and look like tiny flags on narrow stalks. They're more common as we age and often happen at the site of friction including the groin and vulva. Tags can stand alone or have many friends. In this instance, we would prefer loners. Your doc won't bother doing anything about a skin tag unless it's irritating you or growing. But lots of women want them removed for aesthetic reasons. You can get them taken off at your doctor's office, and only local anesthesia is required. Pesky skin tags are really common in armpits, too. *BUMMER ALERT: THEY CAN COME BACK. DID SOMEONE SAY DÉJÀ VU?*

SEBACEOUS CYSTS

Sebaceous cysts are dome-shaped, soft, and smooth white bumps under the surface of your vulva's skin. They're usually smaller than a pea and painless. There can be only one or several. A diagnosis is usually made by your doc just by looking—and treatment (normally an in-office surgical removal) is optional.

INGUINAL LYMPH NODES

We all have lymph nodes in our groin. Normal ones are usually less than ¼ inch (1 cm) in diameter, and they're usually soft and easily movable. If you're thin, you might be able to feel them. But there are instances when these friendly nodes become inflamed, enlarged, and tender. It might be the result of infection or trauma—for example, because of an infection from shaving. Less commonly, cancer or other illness can be the cause. So it's a good idea to see your doctor if your nodes are persistently enlarged.

VAGINAL CANCER

Vaginal cancer is somewhat rare—only about 3 percent of genital cancers start in the vagina, but other cancers can metastasize there. Primary vaginal cancer is more common in women with multiple lifetime sexual partners, who have had intercourse at an early age, who smoke, and who have HPV. The most common symptom is abnormal bleeding. Your health care provider will take a biopsy, and if it's positive, various treatments will be considered.

IMPERFORATE HYMEN

The hymen is a thin membrane that surrounds the vaginal opening—or at least it was. Yours is likely broken if you've had any penetration or even just engaged in vigorous activities such as horseback riding (see page 92). The most common shape is usually half-moon. Sometimes the hymen is too thick or incompletely "broken" and it obstructs the vaginal opening. How would you know? Well, typically, a young woman will be unable to insert a tampon or have sex because "there is a blockage." Diagnosis is usually made by physical exam, and treatment involves simple surgical repair.

VAGINAL SEPTUM

This is a thick band of either horizontal or vertical tissue that may shorten or misshape the inside of your V, and it's a problem you're born with. Some women with a vaginal septum complain of difficulty inserting tampons, bleeding even though a tampon is inserted, and painful sex. On the other hand, some have no symptoms. Diagnosis is made by exam; treatment, if needed, is surgical.

CONGENITAL ABSENCE OF VAGINA

Vaginal agenesis, or Mayer-Rokitansky-Kuster-Hauser (MRKH) syndrome, refers to the congenital absence of the vagina—in other words, being born without a vagina. This is relatively uncommon; approximately 1 in 4,000 to 10,000 women is affected. Ovaries are present and functional, uterus and cervix may be present, but menstruation never happens and intercourse isn't possible. Diagnosis is made with history, physical exam, and imaging. Treatment involves the use of vaginal dilators to gradually create a vagina suitable for intercourse. In some cases, surgery is used to create a vagina.

R

IS FOR RECTUM

Rectum? Nearly
Killed 'Em!

Are we as simple as a compass? Well, most Western women are not. About three-quarters of the population (this estimate is not based on research!) feels squeamish when it comes to talking about rectal and anal issues. Even my smartest, most daring friends get uptight and coy about their backside. But I say, "Hey, girlfriend, what's the big deal? The rectum is just another part of your anatomy. Why play favorites?" And then I explain anal issues without coating anything with sugar. Okay, so that might be a bad cliché!

**WE'RE NOT ALL ASSHOLES . . .
BUT WE ALL HAVE ONE.**

Just like the four main directions (north, south, east, and west) the body also possesses four openings or doors—the east door is mouth, the west door is rectum, the north door is head, while the south door is private part.

—Atharva Veda

Now I'll go on . . . and remember, let's not go crazy about this . . .

The rectum is the lower part of the large intestine where the body stores stool. The anus is the opening of the rectum through which stool passes out of the body. Problems with the rectum and anus are common. They include hemorrhoids, abscesses, incontinence, and cancer of the rectum or anus. If you have any anal or rectal troubles—especially if you have pain or bleeding—don't be too embarrassed to speak with your doctor about it.

BUZZKILL The bottom wall of the vagina is the same as the top wall of the rectum. Or to put it visually: The posterior vaginal wall and anterior rectal wall lie on top of each other, kind of like one garden hose on top of another garden hose. That's why injury to one can lead to injury in the other. Rectal problems or infections can be closely associated with vaginal infections.

IT FEELS LIKE THERE'S AN ITCHY LUMP IN MY RECTUM. UH . . . WHAT'S GOING ON THERE?

It's probably no biggie—although it might be large in size. The most likely diagnosis is hemorrhoids, which are nothing more than enlarged or swollen veins around your rectum. Often they can be felt, or seen, around the outside of your anus or they may be hidden inside. There might be other less-than-charming symptoms such as rectal bleeding, pain, bulging tissue around the anus, leakage of feces, or difficulty cleaning after a bowel movement. Even though there's no reason to be embarrassed, this might not be something you want to talk about on a first date.

DID YOU KNOW? Johnny Cash, the amazing country singer, refused to allow his hit song "Ring of Fire" to be used in a hemorrhoid commercial!

Hemorrhoids may develop because you're overweight, pregnant, standing or sitting for long periods, or straining during physical labor or constipation.

DEALING

Testing diagnosis is made by clinical exam or by an anoscopy (looking inside the anus with a small instrument).

TREATMENT

- Prevention of constipation and avoiding straining during a bowel movement.

- Sitz baths for 15 minutes, two or three times a day, give relief. These warm-water soaks improve blood flow and relax the muscle around the anus.

- Topical creams or suppositories available OTC or by prescription for relief of pain, itching, and swelling.

- Banding, cautery, or surgical therapy for larger hemorrhoids.

AFTER A BOWEL MOVEMENT, I FEEL A BURNING OR TEARING AND THEN A THROBBING PAIN THAT LASTS FOR A FEW MINUTES . . . SOMETIMES EVEN LONGER.

You could be suffering with fissures, which are tears in the lining of the anus. It's usually not a big deal, and the fissure can heal spontaneously. If not, no worries, there are treatments. But if you're freaking out, it's understandable. And if you see even a small amount of blood in the toilet bowl, it can be frightening—because it looks like a ton of blood in the water. Anal fissures are caused by trauma including passage of bulky, hard stools. Or they might be related to intestinal conditions such as Crohn's disease. Speak with your doctor. Often, the gynecologist is the only doctor women see on a regular basis, so sharing this info during your visit is super important. Remember, you can discuss anything with your gyno, even if it isn't directly vaj or boob related.

DEALING

There are a number of things you can do, ranging from OTC to surgery.

TREATMENT

- Eliminating constipation with fiber and laxatives

- Softening your stools with OTC stool softeners

- Sitz baths

- Nitroglycerin ointment or Botox injections to help healing

- Surgery

OMG! I LOVE MY BABY—AND I WOULD HAVE DONE ANYTHING TO GIVE BIRTH TO HER—INCLUDING HAVING MY RECTUM RIPPED APART—WHICH ACTUALLY HAPPENED! WHAT GIVES?

We bet she's the most beautiful little one in the world. That said, you may have had an obstetrical tear involving the anal sphincter and rectum. Tears can lead to chronic conditions including anorectal abscess, fecal incontinence, and painful sex. There are certain circumstances that put women at higher risk for the condition including delivery of your first baby or a big baby, Indian or Asian ethnicity, episiotomy, length of labor, and operative delivery with forceps or vacuum.

DEALING

Time and patience are musts for healing during your postpartum period.

TREATMENT

- Sitz baths.

- Stool softeners to avoid constipation and straining.

- Topical and oral analgesics for pain.

- In the months following delivery, estrogen cream and lubricants may help with painful sex.

- Surgical consultation or procedure may be needed for chronic issues. *NOTHING IS TOO GROSS TO TALK ABOUT.*

HOW CAN I SAY THIS? I'M SOOOOO ITCHY!

Anal pruritis, or anal itching, is annoying but usually just a benign condition and nothing to lose sleep about. Dietary factors and fecal soilage (leaky stool, soiling oneself) are the most common causes; however, overzealous cleansing, hemorrhoids, fissures, skin conditions like psoriasis, or even cancer could also contribute to this condition. Interestingly, itching is often made worse by application of multiple medications and products for relief. In this instance, the old adage "Less is more" might be the way to go.

DEALING

Diagnosis is usually made with a thorough history, clinical exam, and in some cases a skin biopsy, sigmoidoscopy (an examination of the lower colon with a flexible instrument called a sigmoidoscope), or colonoscopy. The best treatments are aimed at finding and eliminating the cause.

TREATMENT

- Avoiding trigger foods such as coffee, tea, cola, chocolate, spicy foods, tomatoes, and citrus

- Using unscented laundry detergent and mild bath products

> *Take it easy, Doc. You're boldly going where no man has dared to go.*
>
> —Dave Barry,
> Humorist

- Nixing baby wipes, which may contain alcohol or witch hazel and can worsen symptoms for some women

- Wiping with pre-moistened toilet paper

- Applying 1% hydrocortisone cream twice daily to the anus

- Applying protective ointments such as A+D ointment or those containing zinc oxide topically

- Cleansing with a moisturizing anal cleanser like Balneol after a bowel movement

- Taking antihistamines until local treatments start to work

THE COLONOSCOPY

A colonoscopy allows a medical expert to view the lining of your rectum and the entire colon. It's an all-in-one procedure used to screen for colon cancer and to evaluate rectal bleeding, unexplained iron deficiency anemia, or chronic abdominal or rectal pain. Preparing for it isn't the most fun thing in the world, and it's certainly not the time to plan a night out on the town. In fact, it's probably a good idea to make your toilet your best friend because a bowel prep, or complete cleansing of the colon with a liquid prep and laxatives, is needed prior to colonoscopy. Right

before your colonoscopy, you'll be sedated with IV medication. And then you wake up! And it's over! Well, it's over aside from some residual flatulence. Most patients recover easily after colonoscopy and complications are rare. Everyone, beginning at age 50 or earlier, should undergo colon cancer screenings, even if they don't have any symptoms. Barium enema and stool tests, including a new mail-in collect-at-home stool DNA test, are used to evaluate rectums. Fun!

I NOTICE BLOOD IN THE TOILET AFTER I HAVE A BOWEL MOVEMENT. IS IT SERIOUS?

Rectal bleeding is common but should always be checked out by your doctor. It is most often caused by hemorrhoids or an anal fissure (we've already talked about those), but other causes include colon or rectal cancer, colon polyps, colitis (inflammation of the colon), and diverticulosis (inflammation of the small outpouches of the colon).

WAYS TO PREVENT PROBLEMS WITH YOUR POSTERIOR

Eat a high-fiber diet. It's one of the best ways to soften your stools. Fiber is found in fruits and vegetables or can be taken as an OTC supplement. Between 20 and 35 grams of dietary fiber is recommended daily.

- Keep the area clean and dry. Use nonperfumed soap and unscented toilet paper.
- Avoid feminine sprays or any products containing talc. The use of talc on the genital area is associated with ovarian cancer.
- Sleep in loose-fitting garments.
- Nix tight thongs.
- Use a bidet, which can now be purchased as attachments for regular toilets
- Wipe with toilet paper moistened with water or an OTC hygienic cleansing solution such as Balneol.

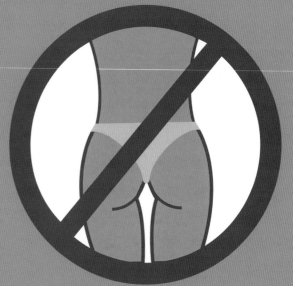

DEALING

The best test for rectal bleeding depends on your age, symptoms, and past history. A rectal exam may be all that is needed for diagnosis. Anoscopy is done in the office, without sedation, and allows inspection of the anus and lower rectum. Sigmoidoscopy examines the rectum and most of the lower colon. It is also done in the office and without sedation.

TREATMENT

This varies widely depending on the underlying cause of the bleeding. In some cases, no treatment is needed and reassurance that there is nothing to worry about can be provided.

I ENJOY ANAL SEX. IS THERE ANYTHING I SHOULD BE WORRIED ABOUT?

On the upside, anal sex cannot cause pregnancy. On the downside, it can cause tiny tears in the anus. That's why some sexually transmitted diseases can be transmitted during anal sex including HIV, herpes, and HPV. Because the anus is so much tighter than the vagina, lube, and lots of it, is highly recommended during anal sex to avoid tears and/or trauma. As long as you take care, you can just enjoy yourself.

FOR THE LAST FEW MONTHS, MY BOWEL MOVEMENTS HAVE BEEN IRREGULAR. IS THERE SOMETHING I CAN DO ABOUT IT?

There's an obsession with bowel function throughout the world and Americans are no exception. But the truth is, one size does not fit all. How many times you drop a deuce varies widely from several bowel movements a day to one every two or three days. Generally, you're considered to be constipated if a bowel movement has not occurred for three or more days. That said, let's move on:

Irregularity can occur during pregnancy, menstruation, and menopause. Symptoms include constipation, diarrhea, gas, irritable bowel, and discomfort. Don't worry. Most of these conditions aren't serious and can be easily managed with diet changes and judicial use of over-the-counter medications. Rarely are chronic symptoms the sign of a more serious condition. On the other hand, if symptoms are persistent and they don't go away with diet, you should have your doctor check it out.

CONSTIPATION Hard or infrequent stools that may be painful. In most cases, constipation is not a sign of a serious problem. A high-fiber diet, plenty of water, exercise, and not holding your stool will prevent constipation. A laxative may be recommended if constipation persists; keep in mind that overuse of stimulant laxatives may cause a dependency on them.

DIARRHEA Having three or more loose bowel movements per day and may involve cramping. Although it can be uncomfortable, it's generally not a serious condition. Certain foods as well as medical conditions can cause the problem. You should contact your doctor if diarrhea lasts longer than 24 hours, is bloody, or is associated with fever since you may have an infection or other problem requiring an aggressive workup and treatment.

IRRITABLE BOWEL SYNDROME (IBS) This condition affects mainly women aged 30 to 50, and symptoms can be intermittent. The cause is unclear but the colon seems to be more sensitive in general. Symptoms include gas, bloating, alternating constipation and diarrhea, and mucus in the stool. You should see your doctor for any persistent symptoms to ensure you don't have a more serious condition. Scary but true: Ovarian cancer symptoms can be vague, but they often include bloating, abdominal distention, and a change in bowel habits.

GAS How embarrassing is gas? Well, unless you're into fart jokes. Everyone passes gas—it's a fact of life. It particularly and sometimes painfully affects those who are lactose intolerant and those who have trouble digesting beans and certain vegetables such as cabbage and broccoli. You can prevent gas by eliminating dietary triggers or taking an over-the-counter treatment to reduce gas.

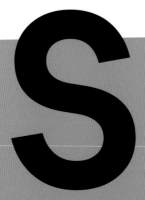

S

IS FOR SEXUALLY TRANSMITTED DISEASES (STDs)

Sex and Consequences, Safe Sex, Spontaneous Sex, Unprotected Sex, and Sex You Won't Forget but Wish You Could

Even though a lot of people already have one, it's not like the latest phone app. This isn't something you want. Sexually transmitted diseases (STDs), which are also known as STIs (sexually transmitted infections), are spread from person to person through up close and personal contact. STDs aren't picky; they'll infect women (and men) of all ages and backgrounds. And they shouldn't be ignored like annoying spam emails. Respond to them. If not treated, some STDs can cause permanent damage—such as infertility, cancer, and even death (in the case of HIV/AIDS, which isn't curable but can be managed and lived with for a long time). Also, STDs can spread easily

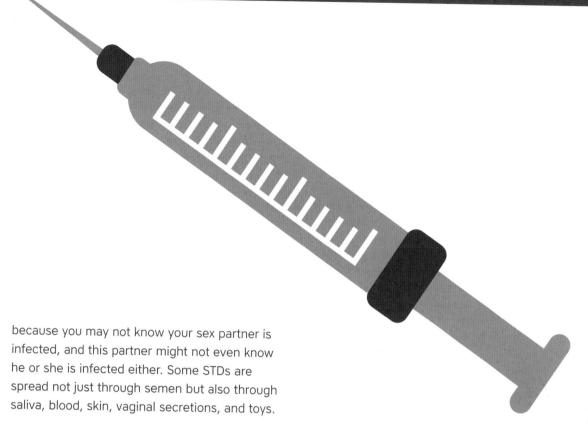

because you may not know your sex partner is infected, and this partner might not even know he or she is infected either. Some STDs are spread not just through semen but also through saliva, blood, skin, vaginal secretions, and toys.

WHICH ARE THE MOST COMMON STDs? AND HOW CAN I TELL IF I HAVE ONE?

Just like guys, there are plenty of ways to pick up an STD and lots of different kinds you can get.

GONORRHEA AND CHLAMYDIA

Even a girlfriend who could win the I-Spy championship hands-down can have gonorrhea or chlamydia and not have a clue. That's why half of women who have it don't know it. "Luckier" women experience vaginal itching, abnormal vaginal discharge, painful sex, irregular vaginal bleeding, or burning with urination—luckier because they get checked out and cured. Both of these infections spread during vaginal, anal, and oral sex—and you don't need semen to spread them. On the upside, you can't catch these STDs from inanimate objects like the toilet seat. On the downside, they are repeat offenders, and you can be infected with gonorrhea or chlamydia more than once. That's why it's standard care for docs to check women who are 25 years old and younger, are at risk, or request screening for these conditions.

DEALING

TESTING This can be done with a swab of the cervix or urethra, or with a urine sample.

TREATMENT Both infections are treated with antibiotics. But if left untreated, either can lead to a pelvic inflammatory disease (PID), chronic pelvic pain, and infertility. ALERT! Your partner(s) will need treatment, too.

> *If you love something, set it free. Just don't be surprised if it comes back with herpes.*
>
> —Chuck Palahniuk, Author

HERPES

Your initial herpes outbreak—which usually happens within a few weeks after being exposed to the infection—is likely to be your worst. So, don't freak out; later attacks are likely to be less severe. The first time, you might have painful blisters, fever, headache, joint pain, flu symptoms, enlarged lymph nodes, and a tough time peeing. Sores can be in the vagina, vulva, buttocks, butt, thighs, and mouth. As if that's not enough, new lesions can keep appearing for five to seven days. But after two or three weeks, you'll be clear of symptoms. It might feel like an eternity. It's not. But it's also not over for an eternity. You can experience recurrent outbreaks, which can be triggered by things like stress, sunlight, menstruation, fatigue, or having an impaired immune system. A lot of women get a warning sign and have symptoms such as tingling or itching before blisters develop. But keep this in mind: You might have an active herpes outbreak in your body but nothing to show for it. That's good for you—but bad for your partner if you're having sex. The virus can be transmitted even without symptoms during vaginal, anal, or oral sex. Exposure to a cold sore during oral sex can also spread the disease.

DEALING

TESTING Diagnosis can be confirmed with a culture or blood test, but blood testing can be confusing to interpret since it doesn't distinguish location of an outbreak (i.e., oral cold sores versus genital sores—you can get genital herpes after receiving oral sex from partner with a cold sore). A culture of the sore will be accurate if it's positive; however, a healing sore might yield a negative result. All results need to be interpreted individually.

TREATMENTS Antiviral medication, oral painkillers, topical analgesics, and comfort measures such as baths, good hygiene, and avoidance of tight clothing. Keep in mind that although herpes is a lifelong condition that cannot be cured, the infection can be managed.

PREVENTION OF OUTBREAKS Get enough sleep, manage stress, and consider taking suppressive medication every day for prevention.

GOOD IDEA If you're prone to frequent outbreaks, you might consider prophylactic daily suppression, a low-dose antiviral pill, to prevent outbreaks and as a preventive measure against asymptomatic shedding (passing along the virus unknowingly since you don't have any symptoms).

HPV

The HPV virus causes genital warts and, worse, most cervical cancer cases (which you can read more about on page 45). It's spread by skin-to-skin contact including sexual intercourse, oral and anal sex, and hand-to-genital contact. But you're unlikely to become infected by touching inanimate objects. That said, recent studies show that even virgins test positive for HPV. These results signal that HPV may be transmitted by more than just sexual contact (see more about this on page 42). Unfortunately, condoms provide only partial protection from HPV since the glove won't cover all exposed genital skin. HPV is tenacious. It may persist even if you don't have symptoms. And once is often not enough—you can get it again. If you discover skin-colored or pink growths, which look like tiny pieces of cauliflower, on your labia or around your anus, they might be HPV warts. Even if you do not see or feel any, they can still be there. Typically these warts won't cause pain or itching. Even though the warts themselves aren't dangerous, they can freak us out. Get this: Warts can occur weeks to a year after exposure to HPV.

DEALING

TESTING Diagnosis is usually made with an exam and application of a dilute acetic acid (vinegar-like) solution that will highlight HPV affected skin. A biopsy will confirm it.

TREATMENT There are several medicines that can treat warts. In extensive cases, freezing, surgery, or laser removal is used.

HPV PREVENTION: THE VACCINES

We know, we know. You've heard a lot of negative talk about the vaccine. But the most common side effect is just tenderness at the injection site. The vaccine (Gardasil 9 or Cervarix) can prevent multiple strains of HPV—and ultimately cervical cancer. The shot can be given as early as age nine, and it is most effective when given to women before their sexual "debut." That probably leaves a lot of us out. HPV infection can cause an abnormal Pap test and, if persistent, can cause cervical pre-cancer and down the road—cancer. It can take 20 years for HPV infection to cause cervical cancer, which is more common in women with lots of sex partners and those who smoke or have a weak or compromised immune system.

A little bird told me you were getting an STD test. Fun!

—Shoshanna on *Girls*

TRICHOMONAS

Be careful what you touch! Unlike the other STDs, this one can live on inanimate objects including vibrators. Women can also catch it from other women or men. Symptoms include a foul-smelling frothy discharge with burning and itching, urinary frequency, painful sex, and bleeding after intercourse.

DEALING

TESTING Diagnosis is made with a physical exam and evaluation of vaginal secretions.

TREATMENT Oral antibiotics are prescribed, and intercourse should be avoided for at least a week after partners are treated.

PUBIC LICE, OR CRABS

A patient with crabs came to see me complaining that her dog had given her fleas. "Tiny black bugs," she pointed out, "are crawling all over my pubes!" I had to break the news: It's not Fido's fault.

You usually pick up lice, aka crabs, through sexual contact, but the miniscule buggers aren't fussy. They'll travel on clothing, bedsheets, and towels. The pubic louse is small and round and lays eggs in pubic hair. You'll know you've got lice because they'll make you itch like crazy.

FACTOID About 19 million new STDs are estimated to occur each year. Almost half of new infections are among people aged 15 to 24.

DEALING

TESTING Diagnosis is made with visual inspection for lice, which look like small black spots that move.

TREATMENT Medicated lotion or shampoo is recommended, and all partners should be treated. Clothing, towels, and bedding used within three days prior to treatment should be washed in hot water and dried in a hot dryer or dry-cleaned. Items that can't be washed or dry-cleaned should be placed in a sealed plastic bag for two weeks.

SYPHILIS

This STD is an ancient ailment, but it's still a happening story. Syphilis can occur in different stages. The initial symptom is called a chancre (an ulcerated nontender genital or oral sore). If untreated, it's followed by a rash on the hands and feet that appears 2 to 12 weeks after the chancre, and then neurologic and cardiac issues—among other possible problems—occur anywhere from 1 year after infection to 5 years later or even 20. Flash alert! In some cases, there are no symptoms. Those at high risk for syphilis have a history of multiple sexual partners. Syphilis can be passed to an unborn fetus from an infected mother through the placenta. Get tested.

DEALING

TESTING A blood test will diagnose the disease.

TREATMENT Antibiotics can cure the early stage of the disease.

I'VE BEEN WITH SOMEONE WHO HAS AN STD AND WE HAD SEX. IS THERE ANYTHING I CAN DO—NOW?

- See your doctor for testing and post-exposure treatment or vaccination.

- Try not to freak out! In many cases, the risk of infection is low. Just because your partner has it doesn't mean you definitely have it.

THE BEST WAYS TO PREVENT STDS

- Practice safe sex! Get tested! Use condoms! Get immunized! Be educated!

- Use latex condoms. They reduce the risk of STDs. Natural membrane condoms (such as lambskin) may not. However, avoid latex if you are allergic. (Spermicidal condoms may increase the risk of urinary tract and vaginal infections or symptoms of irritation in some women.)

- A new condom should be used from beginning to end with each act of intercourse.

- The female condom is available over the counter and protects against STDs. It is single use for each sex act. Female condoms are not commonly used because they're a drag: cumbersome, noisy during sex, and expensive. Good news! The newest version, called FC2, is improved; it's easier to insert and not so noisy—though it's still $$$. A female condom should not be used in combination with a male condom or during anal sex.

- Do not use oil-based lubricants such as baby oil, cold creams, edible oils, whipped cream, hand and body lotions, rubbing alcohol, suntan oil, mineral oil, or petroleum jelly with latex condoms. Water-based lubricants such as K-Y Jelly and Astroglide, saliva, and glycerin are okay.

- Vaccinations are available to prevent HPV as well as hepatitis A and B.

- Prophylactic medications include suppressive medication for herpes, post-exposure immunoglobulin injection for hepatitis B, post-exposure medication for HIV, and immediate treatment after sexual assault.

- Male circumcision removes the skin that covers the tip of the penis and is typically done in the first 10 days of life. It may be associated with lower rates of STDs, specifically HIV and HPV infections and cervical cancer in the women circumcised men have sex with. I'm just sayin' . . .

- Behavior modification is important. Alcohol or drug use can lead to risky behavior. Multiple sex partners and anonymous partners, met online for example, are associated with an increased risk of STDs.

- Let your partner know if you're infected to prevent the spread of STDs and help treatment efforts.

HEPATITIS

You might know the adage "Love your liver, live longer." Unfortunately, hepatitis targets the liver. Types B and C can be spread from person to person when bodily fluids are exchanged during sex; when sharing infected needles for tattooing, acupuncture, drugs, or piercings; and when sharing toothbrushes or razors (due to blood exposure, even if microscopic) with an infected person. Hepatitis B and C can be passed from a pregnant mom to her unborn child. The good news is that it's still safe for an infected person to breastfeed and sneeze or cough around others. While hepatitis B virus can be found in saliva, it is not believed to be spread through kissing or sharing utensils. At first, hepatitis B causes flu-like symptoms. Some infected people get yellowing of the skin and eyes (jaundice). Out of 20 sufferers, 1 will end up with a chronic infection and more serious liver damage. Hepatitis C often causes subtle or no symptoms.

DEALING

TESTING Blood testing will show this disease.

TREATMENT Antiviral cocktails that fight the virus.

FYI The hepatitis A virus is carried in the stool of infected people and can be spread through food when an infected person does not wash her or his hands after using the bathroom and then touches food, a surface, or another person's mouth. Hepatitis A is not considered an STD.

HIV (HUMAN IMMUNODEFICIENCY VIRUS)

HIV is not an immediate death sentence. Yes, it affects the body's immune system and those with the disease have trouble fighting off infections and cancer, but there are drugs that can help keep it at bay, and you can live for many, many years with a good quality of life. Still, it's not something you want to get. You can become infected if blood or body fluid, like semen, enters your body. HIV can be transmitted during pregnancy, birth, and breastfeeding. Medication can reduce this risk. A newer prophylactic medication regimen called PREP (pre-exposure prophylaxis) can be administered daily for prevention. Early symptoms of HIV infection include flu-like symptoms, enlarged lymph nodes, and rash. Infections involving the lungs, brain, eyes, and mouth can occur later as the immune system weakens. AIDS (acquired immunodeficiency syndrome) is the end stage of HIV infection.

DEALING

TESTING Diagnosis is made with blood or saliva testing.

TREATMENT Antiviral medications and medication to prevent or treat resulting infections.

T

IS FOR TOYS

Toys, Toys, Toys . . .
and More Toys

Vibrators, fluffy handcuffs, fanciful whips, nipple clamps, French ticklers, dildos, erotic apps, and cock rings—let me tell you, hot sisters, there's a plethora of sex toys out there, and we're using them. Plenty of women happily share steamy tales of battery-operated multiple orgasms. On the other hand, sex toys can be . . . ummm . . . how shall we say this? A touchy subject—for partners who may be under the silly impression that if a woman pulls out a vibrating penis with rabbit ears, she's somehow indicating that his penis is less than impressive. Well, as those women who adore the use of their toys report, nothing could be further from the electrifying truth. Sex toys only enhance the experience. And on top of that joyful boost, sex toys give you a medical benefit. How so? It's now well established that increased blood supply to the V area keeps it youthful and lively. But of course, as every girlfriend with a pulse knows, nothing compares to the loving touch of the real deal. And there's no reason why one cancels out the other—thank goodness! So, keeping all this in mind, let's explore the merchandise in the toy shop and discuss the many ways to play.

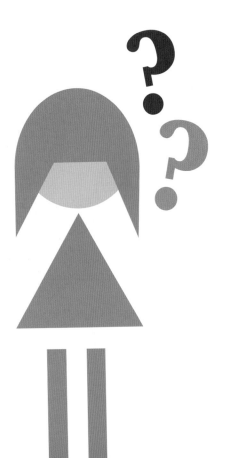

I'M INTERESTED IN BUYING A SEX TOY, BUT TO TELL THE TRUTH I DON'T KNOW THE DIFF BETWEEN A DILDO AND A VIBRATOR. HOW DO I KNOW WHICH WAY TO GO?

Let me tell you. Basically, vibrators are battery-operated or electrically powered (not recommended) devices that buzz or vibe. These nifty items are used mainly for external stimulation. So, if you're looking for clitoral titillation (which most of us need to climax), a vibrator is your best option. There are several different types you can try:

- The egg or bullet vibrator has a speed-control lever and can be used for solo satisfaction or with your partner. It can easily fit between the two of you.

- The hand-free model is held in place with straps that look like a panty. There's also a hot Bluetooth option with a phone app that's all the rage. This option is especially tantalizing for horny couples who need to spend the day apart or who travel a lot for work.

- A simple body massager can be used on either your clit or sore muscles. Note: These are pretty powerful items and are often recommended to women trying to achieve an orgasm for the first time. Bring out the big guns!

A dildo is an excellent choice if you want the feeling of penetration. It looks like a penis, usually doesn't vibrate, and can be put in your vagina or used anally. (If you're into backdoor play, make sure the dildo has a base specifically designed for this entry so that it doesn't slide up where it's no longer welcome!) Dildos can be free-standing or strapped on with a harness. Strap-ons are made in a wide variety of styles, with variations in how the harness fits the wearer and how the dildo attaches to the harness. They are used for "pegging" (penetrating) a male or female partner. Often they come with special features to bump up stimulation of the wearer and her sex partner. When choosing a dildo,

think about the length and width you want—if only life were that easy. And if you're looking for G-spot stimulation, opt for a phallic-shaped toy with a specially curved top. For the best of all worlds, check out the popular Rabbit. It's a two-in-one toy: The swirling shaft offers the pleasure of penetration, while the buzzing "rabbit ears" stimulate your clit.

Back in the 1950s, only 11 percent of the women in a landmark study done by prominent sex researcher Alfred Kinsey reported using toys such as vibrators or streams of water (massaging showerhead) while masturbating. Was that the truth, or were 89 percent of ladies too embarrassed to be honest? What do you think?

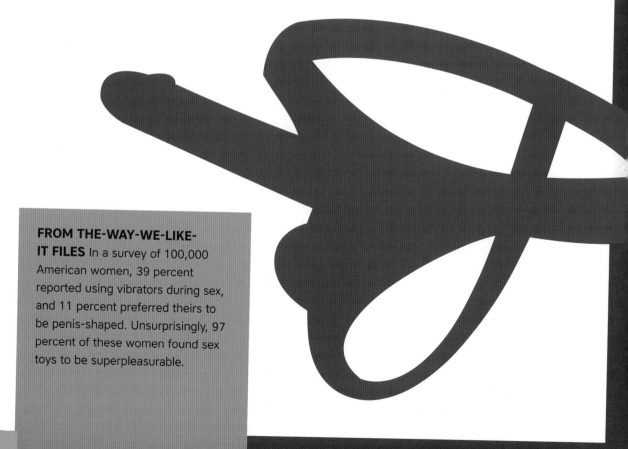

FROM THE-WAY-WE-LIKE-IT FILES In a survey of 100,000 American women, 39 percent reported using vibrators during sex, and 11 percent preferred theirs to be penis-shaped. Unsurprisingly, 97 percent of these women found sex toys to be superpleasurable.

MY GUY WANTS TO EXPERIMENT WITH HIS OWN SEX TOYS. GOT ANY IDEAS?

Sure. One of the best known and loved male sex toys is the cock ring. It's placed around the base of his shaft and constricts blood flow. This may sound torturous to you—but believe me, guys get off on it. Here's why: It increases sensitivity and also promotes a firmer and longer-lasting erection. And they call this a guy's sex toy? One type of penis ring is made of soft material, like leather or nylon and fastens closed. There are also continuous O-rings with no fastener, which can be made of pliable material or metal. But keep in mind, these rings can be tougher to remove and are definitely not for beginners. Another note to beginners: Stay away from metal anything.

Want to share the pleasure? Choose a soft rubbery ring for him with an attached bullet vibrator for you.

I'M TIRED OF MY OLD TOYS AND WANT TO EXPERIMENT WITH NEW ONES. CAN YOU SUGGEST ANY?

Oh . . . where to begin? How about here:

HITACHI VIBRATOR This isn't for the fainthearted or those who are new to vibrators. The two-speed, high-powered wand is intensely stimulating and incredibly satisfying (no wonder it's sometimes referred to as the "magic wand"), so if you like your toys high powered,

then you'll love how hard the motor in this wand works. With its 12-inch (30-cm) length and 2-inch-diameter (5-cm) spongy head, the size won't disappoint. The neck of the vibe is firm yet flexible, so you can easily massage those hard-to-reach places (external only)! For your ultimate satisfaction you can set the speed to fast (6,000 rpm) or slow (5,000 rpm), and the electric DC operation in the device allows for constant and long-lasting power. If you're feeling brave, you can buy attachments for the Hitachi Vibrator (which can be used inside the vagina); these will give maximum pleasure.

THE BIG O! If you're looking for a vibrator with a little more girth, then this is the vibe for you. The Big O! is velvety smooth, firm but bendable, and very long and thick. As with most Rabbit-style vibrators, the Big O! has a rotating shaft, but an additional feature here is that the rabbit-ear clitoral stimulator rotates too, and it's waterproof. The lovely velvety texture means you will probably do well to have some lube handy. The vibrations are quite buzzy, and there are three different speeds that you may have to take slowly—even when set to the lowest setting, it feels quite powerful.

WE-VIBE This is one of the best couples' toys on the market. Not only is the We-Vibe very well designed and excellent quality, it's also wire and battery free. The new updated We-Vibe is flexible and very easy to clean, and has the advantage of multifunction buttons that don't just turn the device on and off but take you through seven pulsing and vibrating speeds. The G-spot vibrator fits snugly internally with the flexible clitoral stimulator bending around comfortably to stimulate the clit. This vibe works wonders alone, but it really comes into its own when used during sex. It's also available with Bluetooth app for remote play.

LOVEHONEY SQWEEL This is the ultimate toy for oral play. It may not look like it's going to give you the orgasm of the century—it doesn't vibrate and you can't use it internally—but looks can be deceiving and the proof is in the testing. The Lovehoney Sqweel has ten rotating synthetic tongues that can be set at three different speeds, low, medium, and high. Even when it's at the lowest setting, you'll be amazed at how realistic the rotating tongues are as the Sqweel recreates the experience of oral sex. Just make sure you use plenty of lube and you'll be hard-pressed to know the difference between a real tongue and the Sqweel. Not only is it quiet, but if you position the Sqweel carefully, you can go hands free.

VIBE REVIEW

There are plenty of different types of vibrators for massage or sexual pleasure, on yourself or with your partner. They come in different sizes, shapes, and materials and can be remote control, clitoral, G-spot focused, as well as waterproof. They can be battery powered or plugged into an outlet. For some women, a vibrator makes the diff between having an orgasm and not so much. Ponder this: Around 60 percent of the female population won't reach orgasm with penetration alone.

COSMOSUTRA If you're new to bondage, then the Cosmosutra soft bondage set is the perfect way to introduce more excitement into the bedroom. The packaging oozes sensuality and luxury. The ties are all soft, and the ankle and wrist pads are lined with velvety smooth material that feels amazing against the skin. What's more, there's even a feather tickle ring, which, when you're tied and blindfolded, will drive you absolutely crazy. The ties can be a bit tricky, but once you've got the hang of it, you'll have secured your wanting "victim."

FACTOID Globally, the sex toy industry is valued at $15 billion, with a growth rate of 30 percent annually. Seventy percent of sex toys are manufactured in China.

WHAT CAN I SAY? GO FOR IT! DOCTOR'S ORDERS!

A gynecologist might even give an "Rx" for a vibrator not only for pure pleasure but for a medical purpose as well. A vibrator can enhance blood flow to the genitals in women who might be suffering from vaginal atrophy due to menopause or lack of use.

Now that you're game, you get to choose the kind you prefer. You can opt for a discreet mini vibrator that's excellent for clitoral stimulation. You can get one that fits in the palm of your hand or strapped to a finger. There are larger clitoral vibrators shaped to cup the clitoris and labia; these types help stimulate the vulvar and vaginal tissues. Or there are midsized vibrators that are often wand-shaped for vaginal and G-spot stimulation. Larger women like these because they offer an easier reach.

Older gals generally need both a stronger vibration and a longer session time. For that reason, recharging batteries or plug-in devices may be better than disposable battery-operated devices.

> **Q.** The most recorded orgasms for a lucky sister?
> **A.** 134 in an hour
> —*Kinsey Report*

I WANT TO GET MY FIRST-EVER VIBRATOR! I'M A LITTLE INTIMIDATED. WHERE DO I BEGIN?

If this is your first vibrator, start with one designed specifically for clitoral and labial stimulation. These types help improve circulation and keep your vulvar tissues responsive and ready for sex when you are. Read the instructions carefully. Then take your time and get to know it as you would a new friend. Know what kinds of batteries it takes. Make sure it's fully charged. And play around. Check out the buttons and switches, speeds and settings. If it's not waterproof, be careful not to get any H_2O near it. Just sayin'. . .

AREN'T THESE SEX TOYS EXPENSIVE?

Well, yes, they certainly can be. According to a recent *New York Times* article, the top-of-the-line vibrator, the Inez by LELO, sells for a whopping $13,500! It offers a "virtually silent" motor in either an 18-karat gold plate or stainless steel finish. But you don't have to go bling! You can get a perfectly practical toy for $19.99 (the Allure) or $39.99 (the Tri-phoria). Other midpriced models are sold at your local pharmacy, online, and even at your gynecologist's office. Still, if you're a truly budget-conscious gal, you can just make use of everyday stuff that you have around the house. You know what they say about creativity being the mother of invention. For example:

THE CELL PHONE Put it on vibrate, and it will give you and your guy's hot spots a body-quivering buzz. Or use the video function to record a sexy flick.

KEEP YOUR TOYS CLEAN AND BE SAFE

- Read instructions before using.

- Avoid material that could give you an allergic reaction (such as latex if you have a latex allergy).

- Wash your toys with antibacterial soap and hot water before and after use, and let them dry completely.

- If your toy is made of a porous substance—jelly rubber or cyberskin, for example—which is harder to clean than nonporous products like silicone, or if you are going to use your toy vaginally after using it for anal action, cover it with a condom each time it's used to make sure it's clean.

- Do not use any foreign objects for penetration that are not specifically designed and sold as safe sex toys.

- Take care not to play too aggressively with your toy. It could lead to injury. Remember that you want to pleasure, not damage, your lovely V. If you are injured, for heaven's sake, don't be embarrassed. Contact your doctor pronto. Chances are your gyno has seen a lot worse.

- Make sure that if you're using lube, it is compatible with your toy. For example, silicone lube should not be used with a silicone toy.

BOBBY PINS Use the pointy end to lightly draw circles around, but not quite touching, his nipples. As the circles get closer and closer to his headlights, his anticipation will build, causing him to get erect. Then take it up a notch and use the pins as mini nipple clamps.

PANTIES Tie your lacy underwear around the base of his penis. The very slight constriction will help him maintain a harder erection, and once he climaxes, the release will be extra intense.

I LIKE TO ROLE-PLAY WITH MY PARTNER AND USE MY TOYS TO HELP MOVE THE STORY ALONG— IS THAT WEIRD?

Weird? Nah. Wise? Well, of course—as long as you're taking the proper precautions. Whether you're playing maid/servant, boss/employee, master/slave, mad scientist/victim, stripper/customer, doctor/patient, cop/bad girl, or whatever other duo (or trio!) you can come up with, props like handcuffs, whips, nipple clips, and dildos must be handled with special care. You don't want to get into any kind of danger zone—especially when there are foreign objects involved. Make sure you both agree on the same "safe word" that will automatically stop the action if one of you feels it is going too far. Read the instructions first before using any toy . . . and follow them. Now go ahead, have fun.

OMG. I'm out and about when suddenly out of the blue I have to pee like crazy. I run out of the store like a marathoner and into the nearest Starbucks bathroom. My pee is burning as if it's boiled water and I'm not sure if I'm going to die from the agony—or the embarrassment of whimpering out loud.

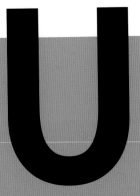

U

IS FOR URINARY TRACT

Urinary Infections,
Issues, and U

WHAT IS A URINARY TRACT INFECTION?

Our urinary tract is made up of the kidneys, ureters, bladder, and urethra. A urinary tract infection (UTI) is simply . . . an infection. Just like manicures, women are more likely than men to get them. But it's not a cosmetic issue—it's biological. Our urethra is short and bacteria travel there easily. Plus, the urethra is physically close to the rectum, where there are lots of bacteria. Most UTIs involve the bladder (cystitis) and/or the urethra (urethritis). The infection usually causes pain, but the good news is that these infections are pretty easy to treat. Occasionally, bacteria may travel from the bladder to the kidneys and cause a more serious infection called pyelonephritis. But let's try not to think about that now.

ARE THERE SYMPTOMS?

You bet! And chances are if you have a UTI you'll know it. Sometimes your doctor can be sure of the diagnosis just by listening to your description of the way it came on and how you're feeling now.

COMMON UTI SYMPTOMS

- Pain or a burning feeling during urination

- A feeling of urgency, or feeling the need to urinate frequently and urgently

- A change in the appearance of your urine, either bloody (red) or cloudy (containing pus)

- Pain or pressure in the lower pelvis or in the area of the pubic bone

- Passing only an itty-bitty amount of urine even when your urge to urinate is strong

OTHER SYMPTOMS

- Feeling wiped out and weak

- A heaviness in your lower belly to the point of feeling pressure around the area

- Back pain or pain on one side of your upper middle back (where your kidneys are)

- Fever is not common if the infection is in the lower urinary tract (urethra or bladder), but it may occur, especially if the infection spread to the kidneys or blood. Chills, nausea, and vomiting may also occur. Urine may contain blood, which indicates that the infection may have already progressed. If you're experiencing any of these, don't wait a nanosecond. These symptoms require immediate medical attention!

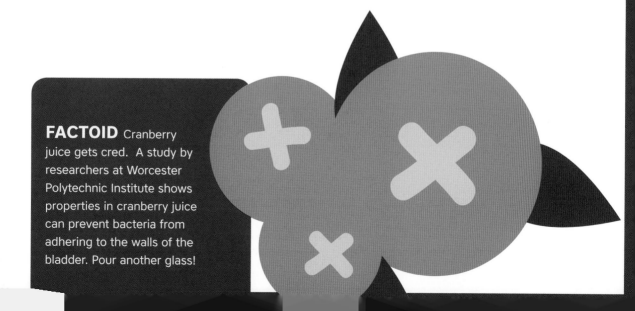

FACTOID Cranberry juice gets cred. A study by researchers at Worcester Polytechnic Institute shows properties in cranberry juice can prevent bacteria from adhering to the walls of the bladder. Pour another glass!

WHAT CAUSES A UTI?

UTIs are usually caused by having plenty of sex—otherwise known as "too much of a good thing." Bacteria near the vagina can get into the urethra and bladder from contact with the penis, fingers, or devices. Cyndi Lauper told us in her iconic tune that "Girls Just Want to Have Fun," and if that means lots of sex (especially after a dry spell), you'll be more likely to get the infection. It's no wonder the infection is nicknamed "honeymoon cystitis." And get this: Doing the "right" thing by using spermicides, a diaphragm, or a sponge may contribute to more frequent UTIs.

We can't always blame our UTIs on a shag fest, though. There are other causes. When the bladder doesn't empty completely—for example, because of a kidney stone—or if there is a problem with the pelvic muscles or nerves, infections can also happen. Those with diabetes, obesity, and sickle cell disease are at higher risk. And menopause increases the risk of UTI since the drop in levels of estrogen cause the tissue around the urethra to become more delicate. Women with genital prolapse— relaxation of the uterus, bladder, or rectum—are prone to UTIs since incomplete emptying and hygiene may be an issue. UTIs can also occur in pregnancy and are more common if you have had several children.

BUMMER ALERT! There's a good chance you've already had at least one UTI, even if you didn't go to the doctor for a diagnosis. One woman in five develops the infection during her lifetime, and lots more have the ailment more than once.

HOW CAN I BE SURE IT'S REALLY A UTI?

Even though you may feel like staying home (or crawling under a rock), you might have to see your doctor and provide a urine sample. A urine dipstick will be used, which is a rapid and inexpensive test to detect infection, but it's not 100 percent sensitive. There's also urinalysis, which checks for blood cells and signs of bacteria, and a urine culture, which detects and identifies bacteria to diagnose the infection. If bacteria are present, more testing will usually be done to see which antibiotic the bacteria is sensitive to.

If you have a recurrent or tough-to-treat UTI, it's a drag but your doctor may suggest more intensive testing with CT scan, cystoscopy (an exam using a small telescope to view the inside of the bladder), or IVP (X-ray images of the urinary tract after a special dye is injected into the body).

GAWD, I NEVER WANT TO GET ANOTHER UTI! HOW CAN I MAKE SURE IT NEVER EVER HAPPENS AGAIN?

Didn't you ever hear there are no guarantees in life? Well, that applies to UTIs, too. But you can certainly cut your chances by:

- wiping from front to back after peeing or moving your bowels, and washing the skin around the anus and genital area well when bathing;

- avoiding douches and perfumed or fragrant genital sprays or panty liners;

- wearing underwear with a cotton crotch;

- drinking unsweetened cranberry juice or taking cranberry pills daily;

- always urinating before and after sex;

- washing up after sex;

- drinking lots of water;

- avoiding the use of spermicides, a diaphragm, or sponge if you are prone to UTIs; and

- considering using vaginal or vulvar topical estrogen replacement if you're menopausal and UTIs are an issue.

THE FAIL-PROOF METHOD FOR PEEING IN A CUP!

When you're in the office and the gyno asks for a urine sample:

1. Open the sterile cup without touching the inside.
2. Separate your labia with your fingers.
3. Wipe three times front to back with antiseptic wipes.
4. Let some urine out.
5. Then catch the rest of the urine in the cup.
6. Close the cup's lid without touching the inside.

FACTOID How deep is the ocean? Oh, I mean the vagina . . . Between 3 and 6 inches (8 and 15 cm).

HOW CAN I GET RID OF A UTI?

Try doing it yourself to start. There are several over-the-counter products, such as cranberry supplements, to help prevent or relieve the symptoms. Your doctor can also prescribe oral antibiotics over the phone if she feels that she can make a firm diagnosis. It's important that you take all the meds in a round of antibiotics, even if you're feeling 100 percent at the top of your game. If you stop taking your antibiotics after a day or two, the infection can come back—fast. If you have a really severe infection, intravenous antibiotics, hospitalization, or urologic intervention may be needed. Let's hope you don't have to go there.

Now that the most common urinary ailment is covered, let's talk about some other potential tract tribulations and bladder bummers. And remember . . . *NOTHING IS TOO GROSS TO TALK ABOUT WITH YOUR GYNO*

MAKE THIS YOUR MANTRA: "Pee before and after sex. Om."

I'M LEAKING . . .

You've got urinary incontinence, and even though you feel like the only girlfriend in the world with it, it's a pretty common condition.

There are four different types, and they are each treatable and manageable in different ways. Some are even curable.

STRESS INCONTINENCE Leakage of urine due to weak tissues that support the urethra or bladder. Typically urine leaks with coughing, laughing, sneezing, exercising, running, or walking. This is the most common type in younger women. Your risks are higher if you are obese, have genetically weak tissue, or have had multiple vaginal or operative deliveries.

URGE INCONTINENCE Also called "overactive bladder." It happens when the bladder muscles contract too often and without your instruction. Usually, there is a strong and sudden urge to urinate and before you make it to the bathroom you've already leaked.

OVERFLOW INCONTINENCE This happens when the bladder doesn't empty fully.

OVERACTIVE BLADDER This causes urine to leak due to involuntary contractions of the bladder. This is typically treated with medication.

WHY ME?

There are several possible causes of leakage:

- UTIs can cause loss of bladder control. The good news? You'll stop leaking once the antibiotic treatment kicks in.

- Certain medications, including diuretics and water pills, may cause incontinence; so can other blood pressure meds.

- Bladder polyps, stones, fistulas (abnormal connections from the bladder to the vagina), or bladder cancer can make you pee when you don't want to.

- Weakness in the supportive tissues and muscles of the pelvis caused by childbirth, pregnancy, a genetic propensity, and aging can also cause urine leakage. Obesity makes it worse.

- Neuromuscular side effects from diabetes, stroke, or multiple sclerosis can cause incontinence.

HOW CAN I BE SURE THIS IS WHAT I HAVE?

There are a number of ways to make a diagnosis, and often it will be a combination of a few of these practices:

- Your doctor will take a thorough medical history and do a physical exam.

- You should keep a voiding diary (a daily log of urinary habits) noting diet, liquid intake, and urinating activity including nighttime voiding incidents, which you will share with your doctor.

- Urinalysis and culture are standard.

- Urodynamic testing will check the function of your bladder and urethra.

- An ultrasound is often used to rule out pelvic mass and/or residual urine in the bladder after urinating.

- Cystoscopy allows the doctor to see the inside of your bladder and urethra to check for growths, blockages, or surface abnormalities.

- A consultation with a urologist (a doctor who specializes in care of the urinary tract) is probably a good idea.

WHAT ARE THE MOST COMMON TREATMENTS?

For some women with urinary incontinence, simple lifestyle changes such as wearing an absorbent pad and staying close to a bathroom may be acceptable options. It might help to make simple changes that include losing weight if needed, avoiding caffeine and tobacco, moderating fluid intake, urinating on the clock every two hours, and doing Kegel exercises (see below). Biofeedback, a kind of therapy that monitors automatic functions in order to train you to gain conscious control over them, may also help. For example, Kegel exercises done with a machine monitoring the strength and frequency of muscle contractions can help educate you on progress and efficacy. For other women with urine leakage, even small amounts and infrequently occurring leaks is just too horrifying and treatment is sought.

Medications that control bladder activity are helpful for urge incontinence. A pessary, a small vaginal insert, may correct pelvic organ relaxation and control incontinence. Injectable agents can bulk up the tissue around a weak urethra to prevent leakage—some doctors are using Botox injections. And finally, surgical intervention is successful for many women with stress incontinence.

KICK-ASS KEGEL EXERCISES

Kegel exercises tone the muscles around the urethra, vagina, and rectum. An extra benefit is that better tone means better sex!

1. Squeeze the muscles you use to stop urine flow.
2. Hold for 10 seconds then release.
3. Repeat 10 to 20 times three or more times per day.

NOTE: It may take a few weeks to notice improvement in symptoms of incontinence.

LATEST TOO-COOL-FOR-SCHOOL OPTION

The new kid on the block is Elvie. It's like a Fitbit for your pelvic floor. Don't groan. It's way cooler than you think or can imagine. This device slips into your vagina and has a Bluetooth antenna that sticks out of your V. When you do your Kegels, it's noted on the phone app and you get the unbeatable benefit of biofeedback.

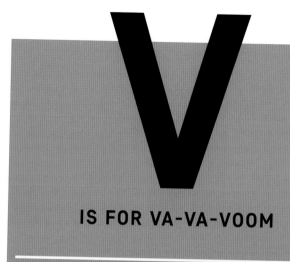

V

IS FOR VA-VA-VOOM

Vajazzling, Piercing,
Dyeing, and Vattooing

VAGINAL PIERCING

Uh, does it surprise you that sticking a needle into the V vicinity may not be everybody's way to go? But if it's yours, the vagina can be pierced in any one (or all) of these areas:

CLITORIS/CLITORAL HOOD This location wins the vaginal piercing popularity award. Why do girlfriends go for it? Well, many say it offers their clitoral tissue supersensitivity when they're having sex. If you're going for a piercing in this region, opt for the hood instead of the clit. Why? Because your clitoris is supersensitive and piercing is too risky: It could lead to permanent pain and nerve damage.

OUTER OR INNER LABIA Don't even think about it if your labia isn't thick enough to support a piercing.

I'M READY TO GO FOR IT . . . HOW DOES IT WORK?

First, find a piercing professional who has a lot of experience with genital piercings. You don't want to be someone's first in this situation—or even their second or third. Your piercer should begin by using an antiseptic to clean the skin around the area that will be pierced. Then a 12- to 16-gauge hollow needle with a piece of jewelry attached—usually a barbell or captive

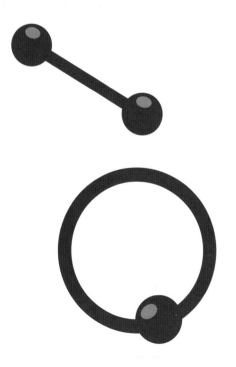

bead—is passed through the skin. Does this hurt? Well, it would seem likely that if some of the most sensitive tissue in your body is pierced, the pain would be excruciating. But get this: Piercing is very quick, and some people who perform and get genital piercings say it doesn't hurt any more than piercing other parts of the body. How quickly vaginal piercings heal depends on the location of the piercing and aftercare. You need to keep the area clean and dry, and rotate the jewelry often so that it doesn't get crusted over and stuck. When you can get back in the sack with your partner should be determined by common sense for the most part, but one to two weeks of healing is likely the minimum needed. That said, a labial piercing takes between one and four months to heal. The clitorial hood can heal in one to two months.

The tattoo attracts and also repels precisely because it is different.

—Margo DeMello,
Bodies of Inscription

REDUCE YOUR RISKS

Whenever your flesh is cut, no matter how itty-bitty, you're creating an opening, and that's just what an infection looks for: a way to get in. You're also opening yourself to the possibility of hepatitis B and C, tetanus, even HIV. When it comes to vaginal piercings, you might also have to contend with bleeding and scarring, an allergic reaction, or—worse—nerve damage. Plus, sex can get painful instead of more pleasurable after piercings. So, before getting pierced, make a vow to answer all these questions with an honest "yes"!

Are you going to a shop that's a member of the Association of Professional Piercers? Will you ask to see its certificate? You can't become a member of this organization unless you have had at least one solid year of experience and have been trained in first aid and anti-infection protection.

Will you pay attention to your piercer? Is he or she wearing gloves? Using a brand-new sterilized needle? Thoroughly cleaning (not just lazily wiping) the area with antiseptic?

And what about you? Have you nixed cheap, infection- and allergy-triggering jewelry and instead opted to invest in pieces made of safer stainless steel, niobium, or titanium?

After getting your fabulous piercing, are you going to religiously follow every single instruction to keep your freshly pierced area clean? Will you wash regularly with a diluted saline solution? Will you use antibacterial soap and water?

Will you dress in loose clothes? You don't want anything rubbing against the pierced area and creating friction and irritation.

Are you willing to give up sex for at least two weeks?

And when you do have sex, will you clean the pierced area carefully with either a saline solution or, if that's not available, clean water?

Will you skip soaking in pools and hot tubs for the sake of an infection-free healing?

If anything looks or smells weird (green discharge or a foul odor), will you go to a doctor to get it checked out? If it's infected, you might need your doctor to prescribe an antibiotic.

VAJAZZLING

The first time most of us heard the word *vajazzling* was when Jennifer Love Hewitt described it in glorious detail to an incredulous George Lopez. Jennifer said she was "crystalling" her "precious lady." Vajazzling is a little like a Girl Scout crafts project, but rather than gluing rhinestones onto popsicle sticks, a professional puts them on your pubic

> *Your body is a temple, but how long can you live in the same house before you redecorate?*
>
> —Anonymous

area using a glue such as the kind used for false eyelashes—more specifically, the vulva after it's been freshly shaved or waxed. (It's safer here because it won't interfere with toilet duties, won't rub off as easily, and allows for good old fashioned sex.) This process is no different from using temporary cosmetic adhesive to any other part of your body. Well, okay, it's a little different.

VATTOOING

Permanent tattooing of the vulva or labia can be dangerous, so I can't recommend it—in fact, we won't even discuss it beyond imploring you, don't do it. (Sometimes I can be bitchy!) On the other hand, temporary vattooing is a fun alternative that you can have done at waxing salons. First you choose a design from the ones available in a salon, or you can design your own and bring it to your artist/waxer. Then you get a Brazilian wax, clearing the area of any hair and making for a clean palette. The vattoo is airbrushed on by hand using cosmetic inks or henna, which is derived from plants. Don't try this at home. A vattoo typically lasts for seven days, during which time you should avoid friction—which means you'll have to think outside the "box" with your partner and probably go sans panties.

THE JOB TO DYE FOR

Maybe you've gone a bit salt-and-pepper down there and want to get rid of the gray. Perhaps you decided blondes do have more fun and bleached the hair on your head, and now you want the carpet to match the drapes. Whatever the case, be careful if you decide to dye your lady flower's lawn. You might end up hating the color, and there's also a major chance you can irritate your lovely labia. To be on the safe side, consider using Brown Betty, a hair dye specifically made for coloring pubes. It comes in five shades, and unless you're a real acrobat, your carpet won't get close enough to your drapes for anyone to detect a slight variation in color.

SAFETY TIP Use a small amount of petroleum jelly to cover the inner skin of your genitals. Be sure to coat all sensitive areas to help prevent potential skin irritation in case any of the hair color accidentally spills. Don't apply petroleum jelly on the pubic hairs that you want to dye.

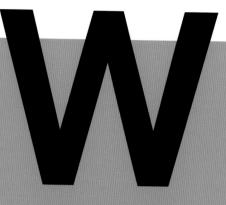

W

IS FOR WAXING

What You Need to Know for Primping,
Smearing, and Shaving

WAXING AND OTHER HAIR REMOVAL METHODS

You think you're fashion-forward by going for a full Brazilian? Well, think again, girlfriend. Getting rid of unwanted pubes is an old story. Indian women were removing their short and curlies as far back as 4000 BCE. In Islam, the centuries-old practice is called the act of Sunan al-Fitrah. For Western sisters it's still a relatively new trend—and probably the result of our love affair for bare-everything bikinis. Getting hairless may not be a romp on the beach, but these days we get to choose how we want to bite the bullet and make it happen.

WAXING WAYS

Waxing involves using hot or cold wax. If you go to a waxing salon, and you're offered a choice, opt for hot wax. It's gentler and adheres to the pubes, not the skin, which is a big plus. Another choice is speed wax. It's soft and sticky and applied with a roller applicator. Although this method is fast and easy, the ouch factor is higher because it's more likely to tear your skin. You can also try a natural technique called "sugaring." It's kinder to your skin, but some errant hairs might stick around. Whichever way you go, you'll have to go back again. It takes only a few weeks for your pubes to grow back in.

LABIA ALERT! Some African tribes enlarge their labia to 7 inches (18 cm) in length using manual pulling and weights!

HOW TO REDUCE THE AGONY FACTOR OF WAXING

STAY PALE. Don't tan down there for 24 hours before and after the procedure—this will keep your skin from getting irritated.

SCHEDULE A PRIME-TIME APPOINTMENT. Your body is better able to deal with pain when your hormones are on a steady keel, which would be the week following your period (as if we need to tell you that).

FORGO A FOXY OUTFIT. Wear comfortable clothes that won't feel tight and rub against your freshly waxed mound.

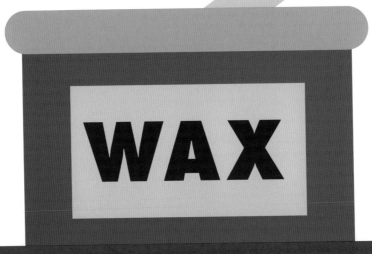

WAX

Nothing . . . nothing is worse than a full Brazilian wax. Well, maybe childbirth . . . maybe.

YIKES! WAXING CAN BE DANGEROUS

You may hate the sight of them, but your pubes are there for a reason. They help to protect our body, regulate body temperature, and catch our natural "scent" (called pheromones) that is produced in our sweat to attract others. Getting a wax literally strips away a layer of protection. It can pull off tiny pieces of the skin's outermost layer, creating a portal where bacteria may enter the body. What's more, the process creates inflammation, which can trap bacteria beneath the skin. Think: skin infections (including staph), folliculitis (infection of the hair follicles), and ingrown hairs. It's hair-raising, right?

OTHER WAYS TO BARE IT

DEPILATION The use of a chemical to dissolve your pubes that can then be easily wiped away. Depilatories come in creams, gels, roll-ons, and sprays. On the plus side, they're painless and work well, and you can stay bare for up to two weeks. On the down side, some women develop a rash or irritation. It's always a good idea to test the product on a small area first. Also, many depilatories contain sulfur and stink like rotten eggs, so hold your nose and use them in a well-ventilated area.

RULE OF REMOVAL Do not use depilatories on inflamed or broken skin.

STYLING YOUR MOUND AROUND THE WORLD

AMERICAN Some bathing beauties remove only the pubic hair exposed by a swimsuit, so how much goes depends on the style of suit you wear. For a bikini, it would be hair at the top of the thighs and under the belly button. This moderate style is also known as a basic bikini wax or a bikini-line wax.

FRENCH Bonjour, landing strip! This wax job leaves a vertical strip of pubes in front, two to three finger-widths long just above your vulva. It points the way for his plane to land. French waxing may also be known as a partial Brazilian wax. Hair of the butt area and labia can also be taken off. When hair from these areas is removed, it's sometimes called the Playboy wax or G-waxing.

BRAZILIAN Grit your teeth and get ready to have all your hair removed in the pelvic area—front and back. This way-popular technique means that hair from the buttocks and area adjacent to the anus, perineum, and vulva also goes. Women who moan at the thought of a total wax-off may choose to have the hair on their labia trimmed. Don't try this at home.

> *A man will go to war, fight and die for his country.*
> *But he won't get a bikini wax.*
>
> —Rita Rudner

SHAVING TIPS FOR HOW TO:

- Nix razor burn and folliculitis. Use a new blade, and shave in the same direction as the hair is growing. Wash first and use shaving cream or mild soap to lubricate the area.

- Avoid ingrown hairs. Exfoliate regularly.

- Get rid of burns or rashes. Use OTC 1% hydrocortisone cream twice daily for a few days. Another option is OTC Neosporin or Bacitracin antibacterial ointment.

SHAVING Razors remove hair to just below the surface of the skin, and if you opt for this method, you'll need to do it often. But forget the old wives' tale that shaving makes hair grow back thicker. It's just not true, although it can cause the hair that regrows to be coarser. Caution: Shaving can cause skin irritation or razor bumps and may nick the skin and cause infection (folliculitis) around the hair follicle.

ELECTROLYSIS Zapping your hair follicles with an electric current. It's supposed to be a permanent solution, but for some tenacious types the hair grows back. In fact, there are a lot of downsides: Electrolysis is expensive, can be pretty painful, and is time-consuming. Possible side effects include electrical shock, redness, infection, pigment changes, and scarring. As if that's not bad enough, electrolysis could prompt a herpes flare-up.

DON'T TRY THIS AT HOME There are electrical electrolysis devices available for home use that copy (sort of) the devices used by professionals. These machines are often unsafe for use by anyone who is not trained in electrolysis.

LASER This method uses pulsing laser light to destroy the pubes. These treatments are safe and effective when done by an experienced provider. News flash! Everything has a downside. Laser work requires a repeat performance with multiple treatments and maintenance sessions. It's a good option if you have a lot of hair, but it's expensive. The ideal candidate for laser is someone light skinned with dark hair. The rest of us won't get the best results. Side effects include irritation, pigment changes, pain, redness, blistering, and scarring. On occasion, hair growth can increase or change texture after laser therapy.

NOTHING IS TOO GROSS TO TALK ABOUT.

PATIENCE PAYS OFF
Hair doesn't start to fall out until 10 to 14 days after the electrolysis treatment.

COMPARED TO MY GIRLFRIENDS, I LOOK LIKE GORILLA GIRL. WHY AM I SO HAIRY?

Well, you may have a condition called hirsutism, or excess hair growth. This affects 5 to 10 percent of reproductive-aged women. Mild cases can be treated with the usual hair removal methods. But if your case is severe, it might require medical intervention. Speak with your doctor, who will determine whether there is a medical condition, such as PCOS (polycystic ovarian syndrome), CAH (congenital adrenal hyperplasia), or, rarely, an androgen-secreting tumor, that is causing excessive hair growth. Take it easy; usually, the cause isn't serious and needs treatment only if it bothers you—which it sounds like it does.

BARE VS. BUSH?

Pubic hair fads aside, I'd like to think that you can make your decision based on what's right for you—not what's all the rage in the down-there department. This is an individual preference. Sure, you'll be influenced by culture and trends. I get it. That said, I have to pass along this information: A study published in the *American Journal of Obstetrics & Gynecology* reports that as the result of removing their pube hair, 60 percent of women developed at least one health problem. What were they? Infections, hair abscesses (from shaving), and bacterial skin infections—just to name a few. Remember: Pubes are a natural defense against sexually transmitted diseases. Removing your shield of hair makes it easier for molluscum contagiosum (a kind of skin infection), genital warts, and herpes to be transmitted.

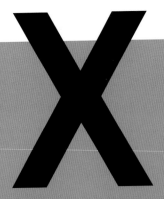

X

IS FOR X-RATED

Exploring Porn and Lots of
Steamy Stuff for Your
V's Pleasure

Most women I know prefer the UPS delivery guy to bring a package other than his own to their door. But what can we say? Each to her own pleasure: Hard core, soft core. Hetero, lesbian, bi. Do you prefer twosomes? Threesomes? Perhaps the gang's all here. Top? Bottom? Vanilla, or extreme bondage? There's light spanking, serious "discipline," latex loving, award-winning role playing, or just playing for laughs. Don't forget (how could we?) cybersex, webcam sex, phone sex, sexting . . .

Simply, as John Lennon reminds us: "Whatever gets you through the night . . . is alright."

One caveat: Yes, alright . . . alright . . . as long as it's SAFE.

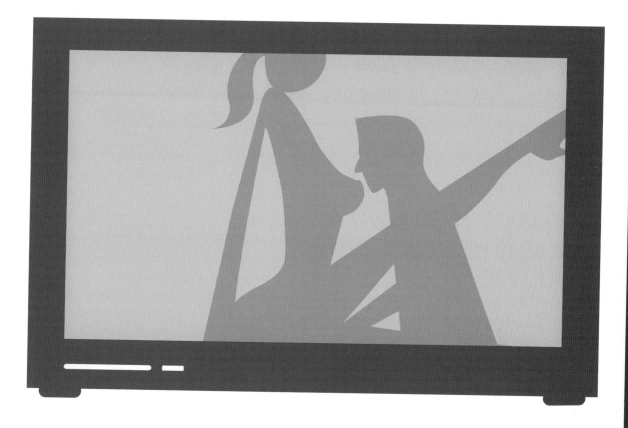

I LOVE TO WATCH PORN. IT GETS ME HOT FAST AND I O BIG-TIME. BUT MY BOYFRIEND SAYS I'M WEIRD AND THAT IT'S A GUY THING. AM I WEIRD?

Your partner is probably right about a lot of things, but, my dear porn princess, he's so wrong about this. Because . . . *ONE IN THREE VISITORS TO PORNOGRAPHIC WEBSITES IS A WOMAN!*

In fact, according to statistics, 13 percent of women admit to accessing pornography at work. Some search terms are divided evenly among both guys and gals, like the word "sex." But women and men differ on other searches. For instance, men performed 97 percent of the searches for "free porn." Go figure.

Want more evidence to share with your doubting darling? In a study at McGill University, researchers monitored genital temperature changes to measure sexual arousal and found that, when shown porn clips, men and women alike began displaying arousal within 30 seconds. Guys reached their peak in about 11 minutes, and women climaxed in about 12. Uh, we're talking like a one-minute diff? Don't be anal—that's statistically negligible.

It seems sisters are also more sexually fluid when it comes to viewing the "dirty." When researchers showed gay, lesbian, and straight porn to heterosexual and homosexual women and men, they found that while the guys got hotter faster and more intensely when the porn mirrored their particular sexual orientation, women liked it all—or at least their bods did.

> *My reaction to porno films is as follows: After the first ten minutes, I want to go home and screw. After the first twenty minutes, I never want to screw again as long as I live.*
>
> —Erica Jong, Feminist Writer

I'VE READ ABOUT GETTING ADDICTED TO PORN. COULD THAT HAPPEN TO ME?

YES . . . and it's not a pretty sight. Approximately 17 percent of women describe themselves as addicted to online porn, and according to some estimates one in three porn addicts is female. Sound crazy? Well, not really. It's easy to get hooked. Here's how it goes: Orgasm releases a dopamine-oxytocin high that's been compared to a heroin hit. Regular users of Internet porn report experiencing an almost trance-like effect that not only makes them feel oblivious to the outside world but also gives them a real sense of power that they might not get outside of the virtual world. The computer becomes their erogenous zone, and the more they try to keep porn out of their mind, the more it pops back in. Eventually the brain learns that porn is the only way to cope with anxiety. The only diff between men and women is that women feel guiltier. How not surprised are you at that fact?

The bottom line, whether you're a man or a woman, is that if porn is interfering with your day-to-day activities and relationships and you can't control it, that's an addiction. You should consider seeking help.

I DON'T USE PORN TO GET OFF— I LIKE TO ROLE-PLAY INSTEAD. IS THERE ANYTHING WRONG WITH THAT?

Hey, what's with all this "wrong" business? Fantasy sexual role-play can take you deeper into another character and release you from the restrictions you put on yourself in your daily life. It means more preparation, and more pretend risks, but the difference is palpable. French maid? Riding ponies? Rubber dolls? Hey, kink is fine, as long as it's safe, your partner agrees with the game plan, and your fantasy playtime is neither hurting nor impacting anyone else. One rule that may not be broken—ever: Be sure you have a "safe word" that will instantly stop the play—no questions asked.

FROM THE YOU-CAN'T-MAKE-THIS-STUFF-UP FILES While the economy was in free fall, a female accountant at the Securities and Exchange Commission tried to access online porn from her office laptop nearly 1,800 times in two weeks. She also had 600 sexually explicit images saved on her hard drive.

ROLE-PLAYING TIPS

Spehd some time thinking about it before putting your play into action. Some people start out a bit shy and nervous with the idea of dressing up as someone else and playing a role. The best way to get comfortable with sexual role-play is to get prepared.

Ask yourself these questions: Who do you want to be? What's the scenario? How can you dress it up? What's your motivation? What (and where) are the boundaries and the ground rules?

DISCOVER A FANTASY ROLE THAT RESONATES Nurse, policewoman, teenage slut, bored housewife, and dominatrix. Find a fantasy that connects with your deepest self.

IT'S ALL IN THE DETAILS When you first imagine a sexual scene the main points may be enough to get you going, but the more detail you can add to the fantasy, the more alive it becomes. Details can also be great for awkward moments when you don't know what to do next.

CHOOSE COSTUMES AND PROPS As adults we don't get to play nearly enough, and fantasy sexual role-play is a perfect opportunity to dress up and have fun. Once you've decided on who you want to be, think about ways to add to your character and role through clothing and props.

FIND YOUR MOTIVATION Now that you know who you are, where you are, and what you're wearing, it's time to consider the psychology of your role. Analyze your character. What's her motivation? What turns your character on, what turns her off, what pushes her buttons or drives her wild? Are you dominant? Submissive? Do you switch back and forth?

KEEP THOSE BOUNDARIES Obviously, we can't say it enough: Setting ground rules and boundaries with the person or people you're going to be playing out a fantasy sexual role-play with is essential. Some of these rules should be common sense and common courtesy, like no laughing at someone and no judging each other in the moment. Other rules will take some thought and good communication.

USE MASTURBATION TO EXPLORE THE FANTASY When we think of fantasy sexual role-play, we usually imagine it involves at least two people. But masturbation offers some of the most fertile ground for developing fantasy sexual scenes. When we're masturbating, we are less likely to censor our thoughts and feelings. Go for it.

Y

IS FOR YIKES! AND YES! FOR YOUR SKIN

The Scoop on Irritation, Inflammation, Rashes, Allergic Reactions, Ingrown Hairs, and More Misery! Plus the Skinny on Getting Smooth, Supple, Sensual V-Skin

Don't we have enough to worry about when it comes to our skin? Wrinkles, pores, crow's-feet, shrinking lips, sunspots, dry skin, zits, blackheads . . . Well, you know how it goes. So it should be no surprise that your who-ha can be a hotbed of dermatological disasters. Perhaps "disasters" is too dramatic a word. Let's say simply "unfortunate conditions" and get to the skinny on your V-skin.

Beauty, to me, is about being comfortable in your own skin. That, or a kick-ass red lipstick.

—Gwyneth Paltrow

ECZEMA

You thought you just got eczema on your elbows? Surprise! Eczema is an umbrella diagnosis for lots of conditions that make the skin inflamed or irritated. The most common type of eczema on the vajayjay (or anywhere else on your body) is called atopic dermatitis. It's often inherited (blame your mother) and a close cousin to other immunologic conditions like asthma or allergies. You have difficulty breathing; now your putang is itchy? Life just isn't fair. Affected areas usually look dry, thickened, and scaly. Don't despair: Eczema is not contagious and there's stuff that can help.

TREATMENT OPTIONS Anti-itch medication, lubricants, steroid creams and lotions, avoiding irritants

PREVENTION Try not to sweat (good luck) or stress out (ditto); avoid scratchy materials like wool as well as harsh soaps and detergents and environmental factors that might trigger your allergies. You can also try changing your diet, particularly opting for gluten-free or anti-inflammatory foods.

FACTOID The vagina and the eye are both self-cleaning organs.

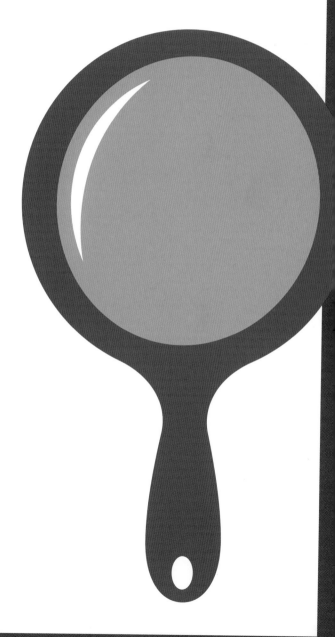

Even though my patients with eczema see their dermatologist—some feel too uncomfortable pointing out skin problems on their vajayjay—no problem! Your gynecologist gets an eagle-eyed view!

—Dr. Dweck

LICHEN SCLEROSIS (LS)

This disease is a real drag. LS is a chronic skin condition that usually affects postmenopausal women. Lose your period, gain lichen sclerosis! It causes the vulvar skin to get thin, whitened, wrinkled, itchy, and painful and most commonly affects the clitoris, labia, and anal areas. Itching like mad is the most common symptom; sometimes it's so intense you can't sleep. Not enough to drive you nuts? Brace yourself: Bruising and cracks or fissures could appear. Even though the exact cause of LS is uncertain, it seems to do with your genes and may come on after trauma, injury, or sexual abuse. LS is not contagious and could be related to autoimmune conditions. Your doctor will look at it, take your personal history, and then confirm the diagnosis with a skin biopsy.

TREATMENT OPTIONS Topical steroid ointments are very effective. Occasionally, steroid injections and antidepressants are also helpful. Symptoms may wax and wane over time and intermittent treatment is needed.

ALERT! Women with LS of the vulva are at increased risk for developing vulvar cancer. Early diagnosis and effective treatment as well as regular exams lower this risk.

PSORIASIS

This is an inherited condition that looks like red plaques (disk-like lesions) with silvery scales. Psoriasis is not only unsightly but also itchy. For some women, psoriasis shows up on their vulva as well as other areas of the body like their scalp and behind the ears.

TREATMENT OPTION high-potency steroid cream

DERMATITIS

Dermatitis is simply an itchy and irritated rash that you get after you're exposed to an irritant. It could be vaginal douches, deodorants, detergents, sanitary napkins, baby wipes, bubble baths, soaps, and underwear elastic— well, you get the idea. It can look pretty bad with red, swollen, or weepy vulvar vesicles or pustules (small blisters).

TREATMENT OPTIONS steroid creams and lotions, anti-itch remedies, avoiding known irritants

FACTOID Are you scratching? Join the 7.5 million Americans who have psoriasis!

HYDRADENITIS SUPPURATIVA

A chronic disease lodged in the sweat glands, this condition can infect the groin, anal areas, and underarms. No one knows why some of us are prone to it, but it's more common in women with acne. Brace yourself: Symptoms include blackheads and red, tender abscesses that grow, pop, and leak pus. Tunnels can form under the skin between abscesses, and scarring can occur.

TREATMENT OPTIONS antibiotics, anti-inflammatory medication, surgery

FOLLICULITIS

Who hasn't had an ingrown hair after shaving their pubes? Not you? Well don't bother reading any further, but for the rest of us, folliculitis occurs when hair follicles become infected. Typically you'll have a rash, pimples, or pustules, as well as itching around the hair follicle. It may hurt, too. But it's not just shaving that can cause the condition; there are other reasons like trauma to the skin, obesity, exposure to hot water in a hot tub or pool, tight clothing, excessive perspiration, and skin conditions like acne or dermatitis. Folliculitis often heals on its own, but if you think you've got it bad, your doctor can make a diagnosis just by looking at it or may opt to take a culture.

TREATMENT OPTIONS warm soaks, 1% hydrocortisone cream, oatmeal lotion or soaks, topical or oral antibiotics, surgical drainage (particularly in the case of a larger boil)

PREVENTION not wearing tight or chafing clothing, keeping the area clean, shaving with an electric razor or a new blade every time (or not shaving altogether), avoiding dirty clothing and towels, and staying out of hot tubs if they're not well maintained

MOLLUSCUM CONTAGIOSUM

Hey, are you going commando in the tanning bed? That's not only bad for your face and the rest of your body (think: dry, leathery skin or worse, skin cancer)—you're upping your risk for catching the virus Molluscum contagiosum (MC). And it's not pretty. MC looks like small skin-colored, dome-shaped lesions with a central "cheesy plug." Ugh! And it's contagious. Even though the skin around a lesion can be red or itchy, the actual lesions won't hurt. Because it's contagious, MC can be transmitted sexually or by contaminated objects such as towels, clothing, or sex toys—or the tanning bed. And even though it will eventually get better on its own, boy does it hang around. If you don't treat the infection, an outbreak can last as long as six to nine months.

TREATMENT OPTIONS freezing, curettage (scraping or scooping tissue), topical silver nitrate, prescription cream

WHO'S HAPPY TO HAVE FOLLICULITIS?
All those hot-tub-loving women who thought their bumps were herpes and got a diagnosis of hot-tub folliculitis, instead. That's who!

I've had patients tie a piece of thread or thin string at the base of a skin tag and leave it there to strangle the skin tag until it falls off. It's a crazy home remedy—but it works and it's not dangerous.

—Dr. Dweck

SKIN TAGS

Skin tags are those small hanging pieces of skin that look like itty-bitty flags. They're benign and pretty common. The reason you get them? Well, experts surmise it's just a matter of skin rubbing against skin. So, if you're really overweight or have diabetes, you'll have a greater chance of getting them. Look at skin tags as another incentive to watch your weight. While they are harmless, and small ones can fall off spontaneously, they can be treated if you don't like how they look.

TREATMENT freezing, cautery, surgery

VULVAR PIGMENTATION

Yes, you can go from light meat to dark meat. Increased color (hyperpigmentation) in the vulvar skin may be influenced by hormones. For example, pregnancy can cause hyperpigmentation in the labia majora, tips of the labia minora, and perineum. The V-skin can also get darker because of a reaction to drugs or a chronic skin condition. And watch out for repeat depilation or aggressive waxing—both can result in hyperpigmentation if your vag is prone to it.

ACANTHOSIS NIGRICANS

This skin disorder appears as velvety, light-brown pigmented skin in the groin (along the underwear line) as well as armpits, under the breasts, and on the neck. It's been associated with diabetes, obesity, oral contraceptive pills, and endocrine disorders, most commonly polycystic ovarian syndrome (PCOS). Your doctor will make a diagnosis of PCOS by taking your medical history and giving you a physical exam. Blood work and pelvic ultrasound might also be done.

TREATMENT: weight loss, dietary modification, taking care of any underlying medical condition

MOLES

Skin moles can be anywhere on your body—including your vulva—and they can be flesh-colored, red, brown, or black. You may just find one standing alone or there can be a few in a group. After sun exposure or time in a tanning booth, and during the teenage years and pregnancy, moles can darken. If they're benign (which most are), they don't need any treatment. However, moles that are growing, changing in texture, bleeding, itching, or inflamed may need to be biopsied or removed to ensure they are not cancerous.

PAY ATTENTION!

Sometimes it's hard to tell the difference between a harmless mole and something more dangerous. Check your lady bits regularly so you notice any changes that should be brought to a doc's attention. Here are some of the more serious skin conditions that can occur on the vulva:

VULVAR INTRAEPITHELIAL NEOPLASIA (VIN)

VIN is pre-cancer of the vulva. In other words, if VIN is not found and treated early, it could turn into cancer. VIN may look like red, white, dark, raised, or eroded lesions. Your doctor will tell you whether you need a biopsy.

VULVAR CANCER This cancer usually occurs in white women older than 60 years. Symptoms include itching, burning, pain, and changes in skin color. Sometimes there's a tumor or ulcer and/or enlarged lymph nodes that can be felt in the groin. Your doctor will take a biopsy to see if it's cancer. If it is, treatment usually involves surgery. Occasionally, radiation or chemotherapy is used.

MELANOMA This is an advanced form of skin cancer that can grow on the vulva. Usually, it starts as a small mole that gets bigger, changes color, or gets darker. Its borders are typically irregular and it may bleed easily. Melanoma can range in color from brown to bluish-black. Your doctor will take a skin biopsy. Early lesions are usually removed with surgery.

THE INSIDE SCOOP ON TREATING YOUR V WITH TLC

Well, now let's talk about how you can treat your cha-cha with the kindness and respect it deserves and keep that honey pot moist and lovely.

- Replens, Lubrigyn, and Luvena are nonhormonal daily vaginal moisturizers that can be used to keep the vajayjay juicy. They are not like lubes (such as Astroglide) that you use during sex. Vaginal moisturizers are more like a cream you might use on your hands—but these go in your V.

- Some girlfriends enjoy perineum massage (who wouldn't?) with vitamin E oil or even coconut oil to help keep their yum-yum elastic.

- There are also vitamin E suppositories that can be ordered from a compounding pharmacy online. These suppositories are in a capsule form and dissolve quickly and easily in the vagina. Note: We're not talking about vitamin E capsules you get OTC at the corner drugstore; they won't dissolve nearly as well.

- I often recommend a wonderful compounded cream with hyaluronic acid—an uber amazing lubricant—vitamin E, and aloe for vaginal insertion. My brand of choice is Sexcellence, and many of my patients swear by this kind of lube to help moisturize their beloved Vs.

> *It's really time for us to grow up and discover our vaginas!*
>
> —Loretta Swit

WHAT NOT TO WEAR AND THE BIG DON'TS

If you want to keep your vulvar skin healthy and moist, you don't want to use chemicals on it or cause your V to be rubbed mercilessly. Down with friction! For garments touching your vulva, steer clear of perfumed detergents, and wash with products free of dyes and fragrances. And don't overdo it: Use just half the suggested amount of detergent no matter what kind it is. Also, stay away from fabric softeners and dryer sheets if you are sensitive. Less is more. Fastidious girlfriends might want to line-dry their underwear. Uh . . . city chicks: Think twice before choosing this option. Also, air it out. Either sleep commando or wear loose-fitting PJs or, better yet, a nightgown. Avoid panty hose, or be sexy and promote V-health at the same time by cutting out the crotch. Strip off wet workout clothes and swimsuits immediately. And never ever choose underwear with a synthetic crotch. Let cotton crotch be your mantra.

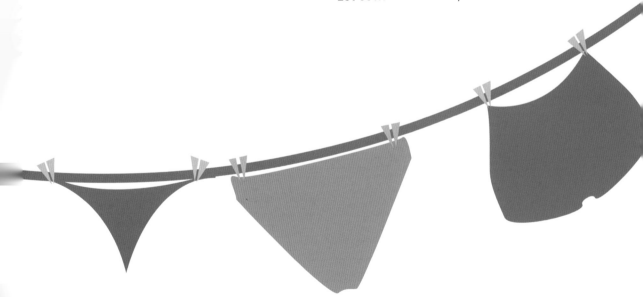

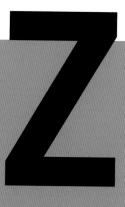

Z

IS FOR ZEN

Appreciating Your Parts
and Nurturing the
Mind–V Connection

Kidding aside, absolutely, positively, as sure as
Kim Kardashian has had nips and tucks, the
mind–body connection is for real. If you have
any doubt, get this: Research into the science
of the orgasm has uncovered that it's totally
possible to have orgasms without physical touch
or through non-erogenous parts of the body,
including the knee and nose.

It's a common experience to have orgasms
through dreams, hinting at the possibility
that our mind may be the primary vehicle for
orgasms. No one knows for sure why this
happens. But just as orgasms produced by
masturbation don't differ physiologically from
those during intercourse, thinking-induced
orgasms appear not to be a fundamentally

> *Tension is who you think you should be.*
> *Relaxation is who you are.*
>
> —Chinese Proverb

different kind. So, I would say count yourself among the lucky ones if you can use your mind totally to climax! For the rest of us, a head trip may not always be the boss, but it's so in-charge most of the time.

TAME STRESS

The number-one way, maybe the only way, to get your mind set to a sexy place is to get rid of stress and focus on the fun. Really, it's that simple . . . or not . . . depending on how stressed out you are. Sex and stress are linked like a chain fence. Most of us instinctively know this already, and get it when a particularly stressful week zaps us of our sex drive. It's not surprising that studies confirm what we suspect: General stressors in our life can impact our sex drive. That means job stress, financial stress, the stress of being too busy, and especially relationship stress can negatively bum out our libidos.

FYI It's not uncommon for pregnant patients to tell me they're having orgasms in their sleep without stimulation and they don't even recollect having an erotic dream.

When we're stressed or anxious, our bodies know it—and our vaginas can freak out—everything from losing lubrication or preventing orgasm . . . to getting a yucky skin condition or (gasp!) closing up, which was formally known as genito-pelvic pain/penetration disorder (GPPPD, previously called vaginismus). Say that seven times in a row! May I suggest some proven ways to chill so that you can get hot? Oh, the irony.

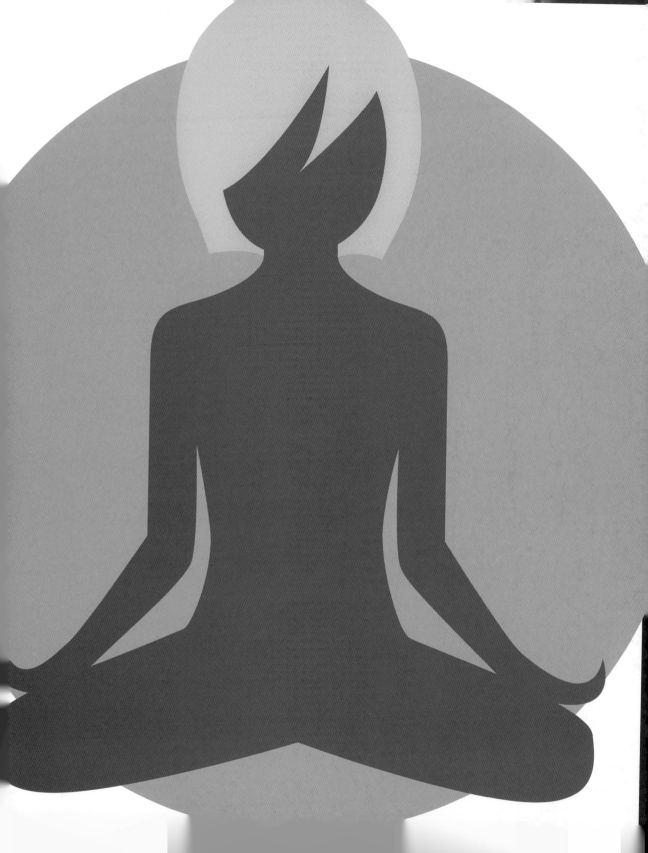

My beautiful vagina is very offended. I'm not offended—my vagina is offended.

—Lady Gaga

MEDITATION

Let's give meditation major props. Countless studies, including those of students, patients, the elderly, monks, headache sufferers, and women with PMS and infertility among other conditions, show that meditation can help big-time. And you don't have to be a heavy-duty Buddhist to take advantage of its proven perks.

If you're new at the meditation game, take it easy and just do this:

- Choose a quiet area in your home where you won't be disturbed.

- Sit in a chair with a straight back. This kind of chair will help you to maintain your posture. Although you want to stay relaxed, you don't want to fall asleep, so don't lie down on the couch or bed or sit in a reclining chair.

- Think of a phrase that you can focus on. Some common ones are *peace*, *ram*, *om*. Don't choose something that is too personal and likely to trigger daydreaming.

- Either close your eyes completely or keep your gaze slightly in front of you with your lids lowered.

- Follow the rhythm of your breath.

- When you breathe in, say your chosen word silently. When you breathe out, silently repeat the word. Keep this going. When your mind begins to wander off (and it will), no biggie. Bring it gently back to your word and breathe.

- Beginners should sit like this for 10 minutes and then gradually up their daily meditation period to 20 or 30 minutes.

- When you're done, just sit quietly for another minute or two and bring yourself back into the room by slowly opening your eyes wider, wiggling your fingers and toes, and perhaps stretching your arms up and your legs out.

- Once you become accustomed to meditating, change your seating arrangement so that you're sitting on a cushion while keeping your legs in a lotus or half-lotus position (feet crossed and on top of thighs, or one foot crossed on top of one thigh and the other foot crossed below the other thigh) and focus on your breathing or on a particular area of your body (like your heart or the space between your eyes or the crown of your head).

FROM THE DUH FILES An Arizona State University study of 58 middle-aged women found that when they were in a good mood they were more likely to be in the mood, meaning more physical affection and sexual activity with their partner.

YOGA

What? You're one of the three women left in the United States who is not doing yoga? Well, just in case you're still in the dark, the practice can free the mind, tighten your butt, stretch your limbs, and keep you a svelte sexy mama. Here's why: You can't have great sex if you're all wound up and worrying about work, the laundry, or the way your neighbor gave you the evil eye on the elevator. That's why really intimate sex starts with deep relaxation, which yoga and meditation can help foster.

Relaxation not only has emotional benefits but physical ones as well. It concentrates blood in the central body, where it is then available to your genitals (for men it flows to the penis for an erection, and for women to the vaginal walls for lubrication and clit sensitivity). On the other hand, when we're stressed out, the blood gets directed to our limbs to ready us for fight or flight. It's primal stuff.

FACTOID Indian researchers looked at the anxiety levels in 50 medical students before and after they started a yoga program. Not too surprisingly, they found that once the students started doing yoga, their anxiety levels dropped considerably. And there's plenty more evidence that yoga helps us feel better in all kinds of ways. Research shows it reduces the stress hormone, cortisol, reduces arthritis pain, relieves headaches, makes us feel happier, and even improves ejaculatory control. Pssst . . . tell your guy to do the elementary yoga position "Down Dog"!

YOGA POSITION FOR GROOVY O'S
Upavista konasana, or wide-legged straddle pose, increases blood flow to the pelvis.

Sex is not the answer. Sex is the question. "Yes" is the answer.

—Swami X

BREATHING

Great sex can be as natural as, well, breathing. That's because breath is the ultimate enhancer of sexual pleasure. It is the bridge between mind and body, and focusing on it can anchor us to the present. It unhooks us from all those thoughts coursing through our brains and connects us with our essential life energy (prana, chi, ki). Breathing allows our bodies to become receptive and more able to form intimate connections with a partner.

BREATHING WITH YOUR PARTNER

Breath is powerful and telling. Without it we wouldn't be alive. When we're stressed, fearful, or angry, it gets short and fast. When we feel loving, safe, and relaxed, it slows down and deepens. This is the breath you want when you're with your partner.

For this exercise, the goal is for you and your partner to breathe in unison. If you can do this, you'll find it to be an extraordinarily intimate (sometimes transcendental) experience.

- Sit across from one another gazing into each other's eyes.

- Just sit like this for a few minutes until you feel comfortable.

- When you're ready, let your eyes drop to your partner's tummy and watch as it expands and contracts as he breathes.

A FEW WORDS ABOUT FENG SHUI

There's an ancient way for you to turn your boring bedroom into a steamy boudoir with the art of feng shui (pronounced fung shway). You'll not only be changing the way your bedroom looks but also affecting the energy around you. Even if it sounds like it may be too woo woo for you, just try one or two suggestions and notice whether it's affecting your sexual escapades.

DE-CLUTTER There's a new study that says when we see our surfaces cluttered, we feel anxious and can't concentrate. This counts just as much in the bedroom as anywhere else. Feng shui philosophy puts it another way: It can block the flow of positive energy in the room. Try to simplify your bedroom and maintain de-cluttered surfaces. You might even decide to really start fresh and invest in brand-spanking-new sheets. While you're at it, get rid of any sentimental reminders of past Romeos.

MANIFEST COMPANIONSHIP It's easier than it sounds. According to feng shui guidelines, some objects scream "one" while others seductively whisper "two." If you want the latter, make sure you have two nightstands (not one) and no solitary candles. And pleeeze, no pictures of you alone, even if you're looking really sexy.

DRY OUT Water is a big no-no in the bedroom because it dampens the sexy fire element. Think about it: You don't want to douse the flames of passion; you want to feed them. So, no pictures of waterfalls, rivers, lakes, or oceans, and no aquariums, either. What about that sound machine with waves lapping the shore or a rainfall? Forget it.

- Next, place your palm on your partner's tummy and experience the movement of breath. At this point, your body has probably already synchronized your breath. Don't make a big deal about it. Just allow the in and out of breath.

FACTOID According to Tantric teachings, if you breathe quickly, your sexual arousal will be fiery and fast. Slow it down and desire will build bit by bit. If you want to boost your sexual self-confidence, make your exhalations long and slow.

- Now close your eyes. Can you hear yourselves breathing?

- Pay attention to other cues while you continue to share in synchronized breathing. Are you feeling more relaxed? Are you happier and more loving? Are you in the mood to get even closer? Are you feeling sexually aroused?

- Keep it going for five minutes or longer. You'll both know when you want to move on to other positions.

- You've just done a basic Tantric exercise!

SELECTED GLOSSARY

Androgen-secreting tumor A tumor, usually in the adrenal gland, that secretes male hormone.

Anoscopy An examination using a small, rigid, tubular instrument called an anoscope (also called an anal speculum). This is inserted a few inches into the anus in order to evaluate the anus. Anoscopy is used to diagnose hemorrhoids, anal fissures (tears in the lining of the anus), and some cancers.

Biopsy Medical test involving the removal of cells or tissue for examination by a pathologist to determine the presence or extent of a disease.

C-section Short for cesarean section, a surgical procedure in which a baby is delivered through an abdominal incision.

Cervical mucus Secretions made by the cervix. Changes in cervical mucus are monitored for determining when ovulation occurs. During ovulation, cervical mucus increases in volume and becomes more elastic.

Cervix The opening to the uterus, from the Latin *cervix uteri*, meaning "neck of the womb."

Clitoral hood Also called preputium clitoridis and clitoral prepuce, a fold of skin that surrounds and protects the clitoral glans.

Clitoris The small erectile female organ located within the anterior junction of the labia minora. It develops from the same embryonic mass of tissue as the penis and is responsive to sexual stimulation.

Depilation The deliberate removal of body hair. The most common form of depilation is shaving or trimming.

Diethylstilbestrol (DES) A synthetic nonsteroidal estrogen that was used to prevent miscarriage and other pregnancy complications between 1938 and 1971 in the United States. In 1971, the U.S. Food and Drug Administration issued a warning about the use of DES during pregnancy after a relationship between exposure to this synthetic estrogen and the development of clear cell adenocarcinoma of the vagina and cervix was found in young women whose mothers had taken DES while they were pregnant.

Douche Usually refers to vaginal irrigation, the rinsing of the vagina, but it can also refer to the rinsing of any body cavity.

Episiotomy A surgically planned incision on the perineum and the posterior vaginal wall during the second stage of labor.

Erogenous Producing sexual excitement or libidinal gratification when stimulated.

Estrogen A hormone secreted primarily by the ovaries. Exogenous estrogen is used to treat hot flashes, sudden strong feelings of heat and sweating in women who are experiencing menopause. Some estrogen preparations are also used to treat vaginal dryness, itching, or burning, or to prevent osteoporosis.

Fibroids Noncancerous muscular tumors that commonly develop in the uterus.

Fissure A groove, natural division, deep furrow, elongated cleft, or tear in various parts of the body.

Follicle Develops in one of the two ovaries roughly a week before the midpoint of the menstrual cycle.

Follicle-stimulating hormone (FSH) A hormone found in humans and other animals. It is synthesized and secreted by the anterior pituitary gland in the brain. In women, FSH stimulates the growth of ovarian follicles in the ovary before the release of an egg (ovulation) and the hormone estradiol.

Gestational diabetes Pregnant women who have never had diabetes before but who have high blood sugar (glucose) levels during pregnancy are said to have gestational diabetes.

Hematoma Localized collection of blood outside the blood vessels, usually in liquid form within the tissue. This distinguishes it from an ecchymosis, commonly called a bruise, which is the spread of blood under the skin in a thin layer.

Herpes A sexually transmitted infection (STD) caused by the herpes simplex viruses type 1 (HSV-1) or type 2 (HSV-2). Symptoms include recurrent and painful sores.

Hormone replacement therapy (HRT) This typically consists of estrogen and progestin supplementation in women suffering from symptoms of menopause, such as hot flashes, night sweats, and vaginal dryness.

Human immunodeficiency virus (HIV) The virus that causes acquired immunodeficiency syndrome (AIDS), a condition in humans in which progressive failure of the immune system allows life-threatening opportunistic infections and cancers to develop and progress. Infection with HIV can occur through contaminated blood, semen, vaginal fluid, pre-ejaculate, or breast milk.

Human papillomavirus (HPV) The most common sexually transmitted infection (STD). There are many HPV types that can infect the genital areas of males and females. These HPV types can also infect the mouth and throat. Most people who become infected with HPV do not even know they have it.

Hymen A membrane that partially covers the external vaginal opening.

Hysterectomy A surgery to remove a woman's uterus or womb with or without removal of the cervix. The cervix may be retained (called a supracervical hysterectomy) in many instances. After a hysterectomy, you no longer have menstrual periods and cannot become pregnant.

Intrauterine device (IUD) A small, T-shaped device inserted into the uterus to prevent pregnancy.

Kegel exercises Named after Dr. Arnold Kegel, these consist of contracting and relaxing the muscles that form part of the pelvic floor, which are now sometimes colloquially referred to as the "Kegel muscles."

Labia In humans, there are two pairs of labia: The outer labia, or labia majora, are larger and fattier, while the inner labia, or labia minora, are folds of skin often concealed within the outer labia. The labia surround and protect the clitoris and the openings of the vagina and urethra.

Labioplasty Often spelled *labiaplasty*, allows for the reduction or reshaping of overgrown and/or asymmetric inner or outer labia.

Leucorrhea Thin, usually clear vaginal discharge in the absence of infection.

Lichen sclerosis (LS) A chronic skin condition that causes intense itching. It mostly affects the genital and anal areas.

Luteinizing hormone (LH) A hormone produced by the anterior pituitary gland in the brain. In females, an acute rise of LH, called the LH surge, triggers ovulation.

Mons pubis A fat pad that covers the pubic bone and protects it during intercourse.

Morning-after pill A type of emergency contraception that helps to prevent pregnancy after unprotected sex.

Ovarian cysts Small fluid-filled sacs that develop in a woman's ovaries. Most cysts are harmless, but some may cause problems such as rupturing, bleeding, or torsing (twisting).

Ovulation The part of the female menstrual cycle when a mature ovarian follicle (contained in the ovary) releases an egg (also known as an ovum, oocyte, or female gamete). It is during this process that the egg travels down the fallopian tube where it may be met by a sperm and become fertilized.

Pap smear Also called a pap test, it is a screening test used to monitor for cervical (and occasionally vaginal) cancer.

Pelvic exam A complete physical exam of a woman's external and internal pelvic organs by a health professional.

Pelvic floor Refers to the group of muscles that form a sling, or hammock, across the opening of a woman's pelvis.

Perimenopause Also called the menopause transition, the stage of a woman's reproductive life that begins eight to ten years before menopause, when the ovaries gradually begin to produce less estrogen. It usually starts in a woman's forties but can start in the thirties as well. Perimenopause lasts up until menopause, which is 12 months of no menses.

Polycystic ovarian syndrome (PCOS) A complex condition in which there is an imbalance of a woman's female sex hormones due to chronic lack of ovulation. This hormone imbalance may cause changes in the menstrual cycle, acne, abnormal hair growth, and infertility.

Premenstrual dysphoric disorder (PMDD) A condition associated with severe emotional and physical problems that are linked closely to the menstrual cycle. Symptoms occur regularly in the second half of the cycle and end when menstruation begins or shortly thereafter. Symptoms are severe enough to cause personal distress and disrupt relationships and well-being.

Premenstrual syndrome (PMS) Also called premenstrual tension, or PMT, it is a collection of physical and emotional symptoms related to a woman's menstrual cycle.

Polyps An abnormal growth of fleshy tissue projecting from bodily surfaces such as the uterine lining, cervix, or a mucus membrane such as the vagina.

Progesterone A hormone secreted by the empty egg follicle after ovulation has occurred. It is highest during the last phases of the menstrual cycle, after ovulation. Progesterone causes the endometrium to thicken and prepare for the implantation of a fertilized egg.

Selective serotonin re-uptake inhibitors (SSRI) A class of antidepressants used for the treatment of depression, PMS, and menopausal symptoms. Low serotonin levels are often noted with depression.

Sexually transmitted infection (STD) An illness that has a significant probability of transmission between humans by means of sexual behavior, including vaginal intercourse, oral sex, anal sex, and skin-to-skin contact. While in the past these illnesses have mostly been referred to as sexually transmitted diseases (STDs), in recent years the term STI has been preferred.

Sitz bath A bath in which a person sits in water up to the hips. It is used to relieve discomfort and pain in the lower part of the body, for example from hemorrhoids or after childbirth.

Topical analgesics Pain-relieving creams, lotions, rubs, gels, and sprays that you rub on the skin. Doctors often recommend these products in addition to other medications to help temporarily ease pain.

Toxic shock syndrome (TSS) A potentially fatal illness caused by a bacterial toxin. It is characterized by high fever, rash, shock, and multiorgan failure. In some cases, it has been linked to tampon use.

Transition zone The area of the cervix most susceptible to precancerous and cancerous change. Also called the squamo-columnar junction or T-zone, it represents the changeover from one cell type to another.

Urethra The tube that carries urine from the bladder to outside the body.

Urinary tract infection (UTI) A bacterial infection that affects any part of the urinary tract.

Uterine fibroids Benign muscular tumors that grow on the inside, outside, or in the wall of the uterus. They may be called fibroid tumors, leiomyomas, or myomas. Fibroids are not cancerous.

Vaginal atrophy The thinning of the vaginal tissue due to a decline in estrogen.

Vulva External female genitals including the labia majora, labia minora, the entrance to the vagina, the perineum, and the clitoris.

Vulvar acanthosis nigricans Symmetric, diffuse, velvety brown to gray-black skin change typically noted in groin creases or in the axillae (under the armpits) in women with PCOS.

Vulvar intraepithelial neoplasia (VIN) Abnormal precancerous cells of the vulvar skin.

Yeast infection Yeast is a fungus that normally lives in the vagina in small numbers. A vaginal yeast infection means yeast has overgrown in the vagina.

INDEX

Note: Page numbers in **bold** indicate Glossary definitions. Page numbers in parentheses indicate quiz answers.

FACTOID SOURCES

Page 28: abcnews.go.com/Health/ReproductiveHealth/sex-study-female-orgasm-eludes-majority-women/story?id=8485289

Page 32: www.arhp.org/publications-and-resources/quick-reference-guide-for-clinicians/postpartum-counseling/contraception

Page 48: www.washingtoncitypaper.com/columns/the-sexist/blog/13118748/rubber-barons-why-doesnt-your-boyfriend-know-jack-about-contraception

Page 56: abcnews.go.com/Health/story?id=117526

Page 74: www.theguardian.com/uk/2002/may/08/research.health

Page 75: qz.com/883888/orcas-are-one-of-only-three-species-to-experience-menopause-and-its-the-secret-to-spreading-their-genes/

Page 77: www.ncbi.nlm.nih.gov/pmc/articles/PMC2838208/

Page 83: *Healthy Transitions: A Woman's Guide to Perimenopause, Menopause, and Beyond* by Neil Shulman and Edmund S. Kim

Page 106: www.maximhy.com/blog/2014/03/05/a-brief-history-of-pads-and-tampons/

Page 115: www.medicaldaily.com/big-o-10-facts-about-orgasms-will-blow-your-mind-305460

Page 131: www.everydayhealth.com/digestive-health/is-it-hemorrhoids-or-something-else.aspx

Page 140: www.ashasexualhealth.org/stdsstis/statistics/

Page 145: www.sex-in-human-loving.com/sextoys.html

Page 172: www.aad.org/media/stats/conditions/psoriasis

Page 181: www.ncbi.nlm.nih.gov/pmc/articles/PMC3714937/

ABOUT THE AUTHORS

ALYSSA DWECK, M.S., M.D., FACOG, is a practicing gynecologist in Westchester County, New York. A graduate of Barnard College, she has a master's degree from Columbia University and her medical degree is from Hahnemann University School of Medicine. She has been voted a "Top Doctor" in *New York Magazine* and has a special interest and expertise in female sexual health and medical sex therapy. She is an assistant professor at the Mount Sinai School of Medicine, a consultant at Massachusetts General Hospital, has served on numerous boards—including the Health Advisory Board of *Family Circle Magazine*—as well as multiple ethics, quality assurance, and peer review committees.

Dr. Dweck has appeared on The *Today Show* and writes regularly for the Ask Anything column in *Women's Health Magazine*. She had a series called Paging Dr. Dweck in *YM Magazine* and has contributed to *Cosmopolitan*, *SHAPE*, *Family Circle*, *Health*, *Women's Health*, and *Girl's Life*. She has also written for the websites Bustle, Buzzfeed, Fox News, WomensHealthOnline, EverydayHealth, Cosmo, Parents, SheKnows, Shape, and Self, to name a few. She was a research assistant for Dr. Joyce Brothers and is an accomplished triathlete who also enjoys sports cars in her "spare" time. She lives in Scarsdale, New York, with her husband, their two sons, and their English bulldog.

ROBIN WESTEN, an Emmy Award–winning writer for the ABC health show *FYI*, has authored sixteen books including the *12-Minute Sex Solution*, *The Yoga-Body Cleanse*, and *Relationship Repair*. Westen has also written feature articles on health, relationships, and sex for dozens of national magazines including *Psychology Today*, *SELF*, *Family Circle*, *Parents*, *Cosmopolitan*, and others. She was a sex advice columnist for *Woman's Own Magazine* and wrote a weekly pop-psychology quiz book for *Woman's World Magazine* for more than eighteen years. She splits her time between Brooklyn and Vermont.

ACKNOWLEDGMENTS

To my incredible collaborator and writer extraordinaire, Robin Westen, thank you for having the **V**ision. You are an inspiration. Thank you to Katherine Furman and Ashley Prine for your persistence, patience, and professionalism in this **V**enture. I thank my mentors, Dr. Kaighn Smith, who challenged me to "do it all" and Dr. Michael Krychman for allowing me to spread my wings and step out of the comfort zone. A grateful shout out to my favorite gyno gals and gal pals, you know who you are; thank you for keeping me sane. To my brother, Stuart, the supreme motivator. To my mom for giving me the gifts of compassion and empathy. To my dad for instilling an undying work ethic and unstoppable drive. And to my precious boys, Zane and Jace, for hearing more about the V than they ever planned on.

—Alyssa Dweck, M.D.

A huge thanks to Dr. Alyssa Dweck without whom this fact-filled, super-fun book would have been impossible. Deep appreciation sent to the wondrous Katherine Furman, who is an editing and publishing visionary and all around powerful soul and to Ashley Prine for her superb, artistic eye. Gratitude to Fair Winds for believing in the vagina. Major props to vaginas of all ages, sizes, shapes, sensibilities, sexual orientations, gender identifications, colors, and cultures. And to everyone, everywhere, who chooses love.

—Robin Westen